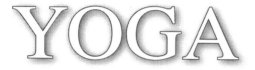

SELLING

YOGA

Ron Thatcher

ISBN 1-4196-9692-0

10 9 8 7 6 5 4 3 2 1

This book is dedicated to:

My Friend and colleague Dr. Purush O Thaman.
All of the friends and family who sacrificed
so this book could become a reality.

My sales job can be incredibly simple or it can be endlessly complex. It can also be at times maddening and frustrating, at others joyous and fulfilling. This game of mental chess deals with the creative mind of the human being and all of the variables that come with it. The highs of a good streak touch the heavens while the lows of a bad one leave you perplexed. The thick skin of the sales professional leads us to strive to find the ultimate path around NO and ultimately enhance the age-old art of selling. This persuasive trade may be the greatest job ever created by man.

Ron Thatcher

FAST & EASY

www.fitnessjobpost.com

NO LOG-IN REQUIRED

www.fitnessjobpost.com

FREE 2 MONTH TRAIL FOR EMPLOYERS

www.fitnessjobpost.com

POST JOBS

SEARCH RESUMES

JOB SEEKERS-FREE

POST RESUMES

JOB ALERTS

www.fitnessjobpost.com

FAST EASY NO HASSLE #775-671-0521

Contents

Chapter 1

INTRODUCTION

Welcome to Selling Yoga. I am glad that you have chosen a career in yoga center sales. The first thing you should know, if you don't already, is that yoga center sales is not an easy endeavor. You will face long hours, rejection, sharking, back stabbing, and difficult managers. But, I can guarantee that if you are willing to work hard, you will have a wonderful career helping people change their lives. You will learn the wonderful art of sales. You will help others learn the trade of sales and most important, 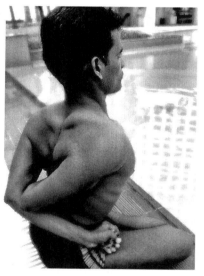 you will have an opportunity to make great money working in a growing industry.

Your number one priority when starting in sales is to do exactly what your manager tells you. First, you must work hard, be accountable, and prove yourself. Once you have done that you can have your own opinion about how yoga centers should be run. Surround yourself with top managers and top producers, and you will become just that. A famous Chinese art teacher uttered the words "the hard won work of the masters was not to be thrown away, it was something to be challenged and emulated."

When I first started in sales, you could either sell memberships or you could not sell memberships. We learned from trial and error. We became better with time, and we copied the techniques used by the top closers. At the time, I worked for a large yoga center company that was just starting to develop a plan of how they would open hundreds of yoga centers. They decided at that time it would be impossible to run a large company with every manager running the centers their own way. They decided to put together a system that could be standardize, improved, tested, and tried. This system, if used properly, could be reproduced over and over and be successful in any yoga center market. When this system was finished and put into place, I felt that it worked very well. But, just as that system came together, large amounts of investment capital poured into the yoga center business.

Wealthy companies had their own ideas about yoga center systems. The system most yoga center companies are using today is a combination of what really works for yoga center managers and what really works for investors. After working for many years and training hundreds of salespeople I decided to work for a start-up yoga center company. This company had high ambitions and wanted to grow fast. I felt at the time that the key to our growth would depend first on putting a system together to hire, train, and develop the most highly skilled salespeople and general managers. Employees that could be trained by us would be an integral part of the long-term growth and system reproduction. The foundation for this system came from many techniques lost by the large companies.

Over the next few years, I had a chance to implement a new system. It was tested and improved. I truly felt that of all the different programs I have put together or seen put together, this improved system would compete with the best. Is it the only system? No. Is it the best system? Maybe not. Is there a room for improvement? Definitely. Although there are many ways to run a yoga center and many systems to be used, they will only work if they are actually put into use. If there is no accountability or if you do not practice, this program cannot work. I feel like I have put together a very basic, easy to use system; it leaves a lot of room for you to add your own personality and style.

Selling Yoga

"You must be the change that you wish to see in the world."
-Mahatma Ghandi

If you feel that everything in this book is not politically correct, you may be right. This is not a book about being politically correct; this is a book to help you get clients to sign on the line which is dotted. When it comes to being politically correct, or helping to change or save someone's life, it is not always an easy task. There are millions of people, especially Americans, who are in a state of total despair. They are not looking for someone to give them a pass and say, "Enjoy the center!" They have eating problems, weight problems, and drinking problems. They are in complete despair over their self-image. They are drastic. They can't help themselves, and they are looking for counsel. They are addicted to a poor life style and need our help.

I continue in the yoga center business for three reasons. The first reason is to make money in order to support my family. Reason No. 2 is to help people. (I have had hundreds of members come back to me year after year and say I changed their lives.) And No 3, I help young salespeople become some of the top business people in the United States today. I have trained thousands of salespeople and hundreds of general managers. Their success is my success. This book was meant as an introduction to yoga sales and training. It was intentionally written to teach fundamentals. They once asked Vince Lombardi, "How did you create the greatest football team ever?" He said it really came down to two things: "I taught them how to tackle and block." Just because fundamentals are basic, it does not mean they are easy. If the basics are perfected, the rest will take care of itself. If you are an old timer in the yoga center business, you may pick up some pointers from this book. If you are experienced and looking to take it to the next level, you may be interested in our first books; Selling Pilates, Fitness Memberships and Money, Get Rich In The Massage Business, and Get Rich In The Yoga Business.

Chapter 2

THE FISHERMAN

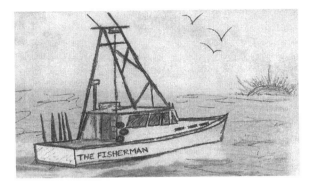

The Fisherman

The fisherman realizes it has been a while since he has gone fishing, so he decides that on the morning of the following day he will make a trip to the sea to try his luck during salmon season. He wakes up early, gathers his fishing poles and tackle box, and heads off to "knock them dead."

"Yoga is invigoration in relaxation. Freedom in routine.
Confidence through self control. Energy within and energy without."
- Ymbes Delecto

He arrives at the launch ramp and decides to go to the bait shop to buy bait. Unfortunately, the bait shop doesn't open for 20 more minutes, so he gets on the water a little late. When he arrives to his spot, he realizes there are many other fishermen already fishing there. He is frustrated with the amount of competition, but believes there wouldn't be so many people if there weren't any fish. After about an hour trying his luck, he gets his first bite. He hastily sets the hook to no avail. Frustrated, he changes his bait and takes another cast. This time he hooks a large keeper; he feels like the incredible strength of the large fish may overwhelm him. He fights and he fights and right when he thinks the fish is about to give up, the line snaps. After changing baits several more times the frustrated fisherman hooks into another large fish, and after 20 minutes or so, he brings in his catch. Happy with his accomplishment he packs up his prize and returns home.

The Good Fisherman

The good fisherman realizes it has been a while since he has gone fishing, so he decides that on the morning of the following day he will make a trip to the sea to try his luck during salmon season. He wakes up early in the morning, gathers several fishing poles, tackle boxes, and bait and heads off to "knock them dead." He arrives at the launch ramp at the same time as all the other fishermen and is the third boat on the water. He doesn't need to go to the bait shop, because he bought his bait the night before. When he arrives to his spot, he realizes there are two other boats fishing there. He baits up his fishing poles, and he is into fish after about 20 minutes. Since he has several fishing poles, he puts them at different depths. After about an hour trying his luck, he gets two fish in the boat. He is getting several strikes but seems to be having trouble hooking up. He decides that the problem may be his hooks, and he changes them. This seems to work and he brings in two more fish. Happy with his accomplishment, he packs up his prizes and returns home early.

The Professional Fisherman

The professional fisherman goes fishing almost every day. Fishing for him is more of an addiction than fun. It is a science. The night before the trip he grabs his fishing poles and changes all of the line. He rigs up and sharpens his hooks to a razors edge. He calls the bait shop to find out what time they open, what the fish are biting on, where they are catching them, and at what depth. He then takes a trip that night to the fish market to buy high-quality bait. He wakes up early in the morning, gathers several fishing poles, tackle boxes, and bait. With blood pumping through his veins, he heads off to "knock them dead." He arrives at the launch ramp and is the first boat on the water. Early bird gets the fish. He doesn't need to go to the bait shop because he bought his bait the night before. As he is motoring out to sea, the cool ocean air seems to increase his keen senses. He then notices the birds in the dawn sunlight are diving on some baitfish. He stops under the birds and turns on his depth finder. He lowers his already baited lines to the proper depth, and he is into fish right away. He is a professional at his craft, no down time, lines are always in the water. He has many fish in the boat in a matter of minutes. Happy with his accomplishment, he decides to try different baits, different depths, and different techniques. He catches several different kinds of fish and is happy to try new things. As he returns to the harbor, the other fishermen are packing up to go out and start their day. One of the other fishermen remarks, "Why don't you have any fish in the boat?" The professional fisherman replies, "If everyone keeps their fish, there will be no fish to catch. Catch and release keeps my love for fishing alive." He packs up and returns home early.

God created man to be successful, yet those who have died
as failures could cast shadows on the greatest of pyramids
because of their failure to prepare!

The Moral of the Story

The example I have described above can be related to everything in life. Because winning is a habit, losing is also a habit. Losers always lose and winners always seem to win. Losing and wining are equally difficult. Losers have to make up for their losses and have to deal with the repercussions of poor performance. Winners work equally as hard. The difference is that winners do their work and prepare prior to the end goal, and losers do their work afterwards to clean up the mess. One of my mentors once told me, "You can manage yourself by inspiration, or you can manage yourself by desperation." Both being equally difficult, you make the choice. The key points to create winning habits are outlined by the professional fisherman. His first and most important habit is preparation. His second is his love for what he does. His third is his commitment to perfecting his skill. Practice makes perfect. His fourth is his willingness to try new things and broaden his horizons. I wrote this story to help you understand or help you to think for yourself. Question: Are you the fisherman? Think about it carefully. Are you the good fisherman? Are you somewhat prepared? Or are you the professional? The whole package.

Chapter 3

THE HISTORY OF YOGA

"Yoga is the practice of quieting the mind."

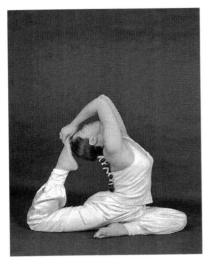

Six schools of Indian philosophy are called "Satdharsañas." Yoga is one of the six schools of Indian (Hindu) philosophy; the other five schools are Samkhya, Nyaya, Vaisheshika, Mimamsa, Advaita Vedanta.

The word "yoga" is derived from the sanskirt root word "yug" which means union. Here this refers to the union of body and mind focusing on meditation as a path to self-knowledge and liberation.

The word "yug" has been later used as the proto Indo-European word "YUGAM," which translates to the Latin iugum and modern English yoke.

A committed practitioner of yoga is referred as a YOGI (masculine) and YOGINI (feminine).

History of Yoga

"Yesterday is history, tomorrow is mystery, today is gift,
that is why they call it Present."

The history if Yoga dates from 5000 B.C. which is supported by the carving from the Indus valley civilization that depicts the figure of Lord "Shiva pashupati" sitting in a meditation posture with crossed legs and hands resting on its knees. From 5000 B.C. there are not many written documents that can be traced, as yoga is traditionally transmitted orally from a "guru"(yoga teacher) to his disciple in a secretive manner. Early writings on yoga were transcribed on fragile palm leaves that were easily damaged, destroyed or lost.

Yoga's long running history can be divided into four main periods of innovation and development. They are:

1. Verdic period
2. Pre-classicial period
3. Classical period
4. Post-classical period

Verdic Period

The existing ancient texts of Vedas marks this period more specifically. The Vedas is the sacred scripture of Brahmanism; which has a collection of hymns which praised a divine power. That first known written reference to yoda is in the "Rig Veda," estimated to be at least 3,500 years old. The Sanskrit word "veda" means knowledge, and "rig" means praise. Thus, Rig Vedas are a collection of hymns that are in Praise of a higher power. Three other vedas are "Yayur Veda"(knowledge of sacrifice), "Sama Veda" (knowledge of chants), "Atharvana Veda"(knowledge of atharvana).

Yogic teachings found in Vedas are called Verdic Yoga, which can also be called Archaic Yoga, as people believed in a ritualistic way of life. During this period, verdic yoga taught the common people to conduct rituals, sacrifices and ceremonies as a means to connect them to the spiritual world. Rishis and Verdic yogis practice meditation in a secluded place like a forest and were blessed with the vision of supreme reality. Their hymns speak of their marvelous intuition.

Pre-classical Yoga

Yoga was slowly refined and developed by Verdic priests in later 2000 B.C, who documented their practices and beliefs in the "Upanishads." Upanishads are the Gnostic texts of yoga which contains a huge work of 200 scriptures that describes the inner vision of reality resulting from devotion to Brahman. Upanishads further explain the teachings of the Vedas as three main subjects: 1. The ultimate Reality (Brahman)/Supreme soul; 2. The transcendental self (Atman) soul; 3. The relationship between Brahman and Atman, supreme soul and soul.

> *"Yoga is the perfect practice that makes the man perfect."*
> -Bhagand Geeta

During the sixth century B.C., Buddha started teaching Buddhism, which stresses the importance of meditation and the practice of physical postures. Siddharta Gautana, the first Buddhist to study yoga, achieved enlightenment.

Later, around 500 B.C, "Bhagarad – Gita" or "song of Lord" was written and this is currently the oldest known scripture. Bhagarad Gita consists of four branches of yoga:

1. "Karma Yoga" — Yoga of action
2. "Jnana Yoga" — Yoga of knowledge
3. "Bhakti Yoga" — Yoga of devotion of God
4. "Raya Yoga" — Yoga of Meditation

The central teaching of the Gita is:

"NISKAMA KARMA HI YOGA" which means yoga is the action without any expectation, that teaches us to do our duty and not expect the fruit of action.

Thus, from the Verdic period Upanishads took the idea of ritual sacrifice from the Vedas and internalized it. Further Bhagarid Gita builds on and incorporates the doctrines found in the Upanishads.

Classical Period

The classical period is marked by another creation – "the yoga sutras of Patanyali," which was written by Maharishi Patanyali around the second century. "Yoga Sutras of Patanyali" is a book of 196 aphorisms complied together that expound upon the Raja Yoga, the path of meditation. Patanyali organized the practice of yoga into an "Eight Limbed Path" called "Astanga Yoga," as the practical path towards attainment of enlightenment or "Samadhi." Hence Patanyali is called the "Father of Yoga." The eight-limbed concept became an authoritative feature of Raja yoga which is often called "Classical Yoga." Patanyali's eight limbs of yoga practices are:

1. **"Yama"** means social restraints

2. **"Niyama"** means personal observance

3. **"Asanas"** means physical postures

4. **"Pranayama"** means controlling of breathing

5. **"Pratyahara"** means senses withdrawal in preparation

6. **"Dharana"** means concentration on a single object

7. **"Dhyana"** means meditation

8. **"Samadhi"** means super-conscious state of enlightenment

According to Patanyali yoga is the cessation/controlling of mind, and Patanyali believed that each individual is a composite of matter ("Prakriti") and spirit ("Pususha"). He further believed that the two must be separated in order to cleanse the spirit, a stark contrast to Verdic and pre-classical yoga that signify the union of body and spirit.

Patanyali's concept was so dominant for several centuries that some yogis focused exclusively on meditation and neglected their Asanas. It was only later that the belief of the body as a temple was rekindled and attention to the importance of the Asana was revived. This time, yogis attempted to use yoga techniques to change the body and make it immortal.

Post Classical Period

A few centuries after Patanyali, yoga masters created a system of practices designed to rejuvenate the body and prolong life. They rejected the teachings of ancient redas and embraced the physical body as the means to achieve enlightenment.

Yoga practioners developed "Tantra Yoga," with radical techniques to cleanse the body and mind, to break the knots that bind us to our physical existence. This exploration of these physical-spiritual connections and body centered practices led to the creation of "Hatha-Yoga," which is yoga for the physical body.

Hatha Yoga is a system introduced by Swami Swatmarama, a yogic sage of the 15th century in India, and incorporates the book "HATHA YOGA PRADIPIKA." The word "HATHA"comes from the Sanskirt terms "Ha" meaning "Sun" and "Tha" meanng "moon." Thus Hatha Yoga is known as the branch of yoga that unites pairs of opposites referring to the positive (sun) and negative (moon) currents in the system.

The existing book of Hatha Yoga, the *Hatha Yoga Pradipika,* marks the nature of the post-classical period which mainly focuses on Asanas (postures), Pranayama (breathing techniques), and Kriyas (cleansing technique).

Thus, post classical yoga affirms the teachings of redanta, that there is ultimate unity of everything in the cosmos and yogis began to probe into the hidden powers of the body.

Modern Yoga

The period of the modern era began with the Congress of Religions held in Chicago in 1893. Modern yoga arrived in the United States during the late 1800's. It was at this congress that Swami Vivekananda, a disciple of Saint Ramakrishna, made a lasting impression on the American public and taught them Yoga and Vedanta.

After Swami Vivekanada, the next popular teacher in the west was Paramahansa Yogananda who arrived in Boston in 1920. He later established the self-realization fellowship in Los Angeles. He wrote the famous "Autobiography of a Yogi" and his teachings are called the Yogananda Teachings. Later Paul Brunton introduced Ramana Maharishi to western seekers, and wrote a book called "A search in Secret India."

Yoga was introduced to the west during late 19th century. It was first studied as part of Eastern philosophy and began as a movement for health and vegetarianism around the 1930's.

In the Mid-1960's Maharishi Mahes Yogi introduced "Transcendental Meditation" to the west. He was also associated with the Beatles. In 1965, Shrila Prabhupada came to the United States and founded the International Society for Krishna consciousness (IS-KON). He spread the movement of Bhakti Yoga.

One of the most prominent yoga gurus was the Himalayan Master, Swami Sivananda. He served as a doctor in Malaysia and opened yoga schools in America and Europe. He wrote more than 200 books on yoga and philosophy. His famous disciple was Swami Vishnudevananda, who wrote the book "Complete Illustrated Book of Yoga." Other masters are Swami Satyananda, Swami Sivananda Radha, Swami Satyananda and Swami Chidananda. Bhagawan Rayneesh, also known as Osho, was a widely popular guru in the 1970's and 1980's.

Swami Satchitananda introduced the chanting of mantras and other yoga techniques to Woodstock. Swami Sivanandha Radha explored the connection between yoga and psychology. Yogi Bhayan started teaching Kundalini Yoga in the 1970's.

The great Sri Krishnamacharya taught Viniyoga Hatha Yoga. This tradition of Viniyoga Hatha Yoga is continued by his son, Desikarchayen and Desikas's brother-in-law, B.K.S. Iyengas. Sathya Sai Baba is the living yoga master of today whom millions of people all over the world throngto . He is called the "man of miracles."

Thus the previous eras saw yogis laying emphasis only on meditation and contemplation. Their goal was to shed their mortal coils and merge with the infinite. But later, the father of yoga Patanyali introduced the connection of body and mind in the 2nd century. Succeeding yoga masters designed advanced yogic practices and other systems of yoga from India, which is rightly called the "Land of Yoga." This advancement led to the development of Hatha yoga by Shri Krishnamachrya (1888-1980), and his successors like T.K.V. Desikachar to discover "Viniyoga," B.K.S. Iyengar who founded "Iyengar Yoga" and Shri K. Patthabik Jois who developed "Astanga Yoga."

The styles may vary but the aim of practicing yoga is to achieve physical, mental and spiritual well-being.

"Yoga is the action without any expectation." -Bhagavid Geeta

Chapter 4

HOW THE SYSTEM WORKS

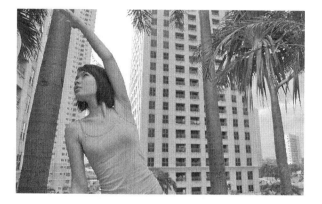

The system works through constant repetition. It works through systematic improvement through practice. The system works because you always have proven techniques to go back to as a reference. Different areas of your arsenal must be trained on, must be perfected, and must be used over and over in a real life situation (role-playing). The system must be used, not read. When teaching systems, I never stand up and tell my staff how to use the system. I make them show me in a role-playing situation, to prove to me how to use the scripts and training. I ask them to present to me the one-on-one yoga package as if I am a real prospect. I make them do the presentation in front of a large group of people. If they can do it in front of the whole sales staff, they can do it in front of a guest or several guests.

I also hold them accountable to have the scripts memorized by a certain date. If they do not have memorized by a specific date I set forth, then I make them present it to me every day until they do.

Remember, the accountability factor is the key to manage the yoga center and yourself simultaneously. Nothing will be accomplished without accountability. Salespeople will not do their planners or use the master appointment book if it is not checked every day. You have to turn any system you implement in your yoga center into a habit. Once something is a habit, it becomes easier and is enjoyable. This can only happen through accountability.

Chapter 5

SALES PLANNER

OR DAILY PLANNER

A sales planner is an effective tool used by most sales organizations in recent years. Much like personal daily planners, it helps us organize our busy schedules. It provides management and the sales counselor with a way to track production. It helps in important areas including the following: time management, guest tracking, personal pay check tracking, prospect tracking, and business associations, personal and work to do lists, and missed guest and future appointments. The sales planner is divided into different sections that help group together information in one easily accessible area. Most sales planners will have training materials in the front of the planner. This is where we keep our scripts and other materials that we have previously applied or used.

The next section of the sales planner provides daily sheets for appointments, a daily to-do list, and sales projections. In the back of the planner, there is normally an area to track missed guests, appointment no-shows, renewals, lead boxes, business leads, and, most important, your paycheck and closed sales. An explanation of each important item is listed below.

If you fail to plan, you plan to fail

17

Training Materials

Training materials should be in the front of your planner and should be used as much as possible. As covered in Chapter 3, I prefer my employees to memorize different scripts for different situations. Memorizing these various scripts is the first thing a new sales counselor should do. If you can not memorize the 20 or so pages of script, you should do nothing else until you perfect that area of your arsenal. If you do not know how to take a telephone inquiry (TI), if you do not know how to present the yoga class agenda or how to set up a take over (TO), you should be practicing in these areas before taking a guest. Once these scripts are memorized, such as the introduction, then these training materials will be used as a reference and training tool. It sounds like a lot of work, but believe me it makes the job easier and more profitable.

Once a month during the production meeting, you should train in each area by the book. If you do this, your sales skills will remain sharp and you will have the ability to learn and grow. Remember the yoga industry is a rapidly growing business. Change is essential in helping to improve the yoga industry, so if certain areas of training are not working or you are not getting better, you have to improve the training information you are using.

Daily Sheets: To-Do List, Goal and Projections, Appointments

I found that the personal to-do list is a simple and effective tool that has been used for years by everyone from the common housewife to the president of the United States. It's simple when you think of something that is important write it down. This will put it on your priority list. It limits mistakes and leaves your mind free to think of other things. As you accomplish each task, you cross it off your to-do list. Things that are not accomplished are circled and placed on the next day's to-do list. This can be an effective habit. I find that people who use this simple tool are more efficient, make fewer mistakes, and get more accomplished. Although this is your business planner, personal matters can still be taken care of at work. It is okay to list personal matters on your to-do list.

Goals and projections should be updated daily. This is the most effective way of learning how your production can affect your numbers. As the old saying goes, "the numbers do not lie." This is especially true in our business. The numbers tell us what we are doing right and what we are doing wrong. The numbers are our guides to success. They will teach you what happens to your numbers when you have a bad day, and they will teach you what happens to your numbers when you have a good day. What happens to your numbers when you are not set up for that day? What happens to your paycheck when you hit your goals? I bet you can answer those questions for yourself. Having an organized "Goals and Projections" section in your planner will show you what you have to do daily; it gives you the ability to control your numbers more consistently and will offer you a daily affirmation of your goals. I prefer to track every area of sales separately. Within each area, I have five steps:

Gross Sales: goal, last day worked, month to date, projection, and percentage

EFT: goal, last day worked, month to date, projection, percentage

One-on-one yoga: goal, last day worked, month to date, projection, percentage

Supplements: goal, last day worked, month to date, projection, and percentage

Retail: goal, last day worked, month to date, projection, percentage

Other goals: last day worked, month to date, projection, percentage

If kept updated consistently and correctly, these areas will keep us more organized and help increase our sales. We begin by setting goals and then use our materials to project our progress as we go along. Each month you should set goals based on the previous month's performance. Like most successful salespeople, your sales goal should increase each month, as your ability to hit these goals increases. As your skills increase, your comfort level and confidence increase enabling you to achieve higher goals. I personally never set goals that are too easy to achieve. At the same time, I never set goals that are impossible to achieve. You want the goal to be lofty enough to motivate you but not so high that you can never reach it. The goal should be in line with what you want your paycheck to be. If you set a goal that is $200,000 in sales, and your commission is 10 percent, that equals $20,000 commission, before taxes. You cannot expect to bring home a $30,000 paycheck. The first goal that should be set is what you want your income to be. Based on that, you can calculate how much you need to sell. You now have your goal.

For Example:

Your desired income is $50,000	50,000
Your commission from each sale is 10%	x10
You must sell	$500,000

Being able to meet your goals will make you a highly effective businessperson, and you will be able to control your financial destiny. The sky is the limit! The last day worked is what you sold the last day in each area. The month to date is a running total; it represents the updated total amount you have sold up to that date for the month. Your projection is the month to date divided by the days gone by, times the total days in the month. The percentage is your projection divided by your goal.

For Example for Projection:

Ex: month to date   divided by days gone by.

   x

Total days in the month. = Projection

It is the second day of a 30-day month. Yesterday you sold $2,000 in gross sales. Your month to date is $2,000. One day has gone by, and so you divide 2000 by 1 times 30 days in the month. It means that the total amount you are projecting is $60,000. Divide that by your goal of $70,000. You are at 86 percent of your goal.

For example:

Ex: 2,000 x 30

$$\underline{1 = 60,000} = \textbf{86\%}$$

70,000

You now have 29 days left in the month to reach your goal. Since you sold $2,000 on the first day of the month, you now have only $68,000 left to reach your goal. In order to find your daily goal you must minus your month to date, from your goal and divide by how many days are left in the month. The numbers show that you must sell an average of $2,344 per day for the rest of the month to achieve 100 percent of your original goal.

For example:

Ex: 70,000 $\underline{68,000} = \textbf{\$2,344}$

          - 2,000 29

          68,000

Updating your statistics is something that should be done every day. You should make this a strict habit, and it should be the first thing you do every morning after you walk through the studio. The numbers, good or bad will show you the areas that you have to focus on for that day. They also show the areas that you are doing well in and the areas you need to improve.

Finally, your daily appointment sheets will have areas for all important appointment information. Each day's sheet will have sections for recording the time of the appointment, for conformation, for how the prospect heard about the studio, the person's name, their work and home telephone number, a note about the appointment, and finally, the outcome.

The **time** section is for what time you are scheduling the appointment. You write the person's information next to the time they are expected for their appointment. The **confirmation** box will let you make a note if the appointment has been confirmed. Listed below are the letters you should use to put in the various boxes.

For Example:

C for confirmed appointments; **LM** for left message; **NA** for no answer; **B** for line is busy; and **CB** for you are going to call back at a later time.

The source is how the person heard about the studio.

For Example:

S for sign; **YP** for yellow pages; **BR** for buddy referral; **Pass** for Pass; **NP** for newspaper; **TV** for television; and **RD** for radio.

For **name**, you should have the person's first and last name and always ask if the person will be coming alone or if they want to bring friends or family along with them. Get as many first and last names as possible.

In the **telephone number** section, you should always get home and work telephone numbers, even cell phone or pager numbers if possible. The more numbers you have the better chance you have to contact and confirm an appointment with your guest. I have seen so many salespeople talk to a person that is calling from work and they only get their work telephone number and make an appointment for a weekend, then try to confirm the appointment Saturday morning when the person is not at work. Since the work telephone number is the only number the yoga counselor has, they have no way of contacting them. Thousands of sales are lost because of this simple mistake, which can become a costly habit.

The **notes** section will help you remember important information you discuss on the telephone with the perspective members. These simple notes include their goals, their problems, names of friends and family, if they are sick, and other key information that will help you serve your guest once they come into the studio.

For example, I talk to Mary on the telephone. She tells me that she was sick on the day of her original appointment, so she will not be able to come into the studio until Saturday. Then she tells me that her daughter, Tracy, has a soccer game Saturday morning and will not be able to come in until the afternoon. She continues to tell me that her car is in the shop, so she will have to pick it up on Friday night, leaving that day out as a potential appointment. Saturday at one o'clock, Mary and her daughter come into the studio and ask for me. I come to the front desk, and I say:

How are you Mary? My name is Ron. What I would like to do is take a moment of your time to find out what you are looking to accomplish, take you on a tour of our incredible facility, and go over our different membership options. Sound fair? This must be your daughter, Tracy. Tracy, did you win your soccer game? Tracy says: Yes, we did. I then ask: *Mary, I hope you are feeling better, are you over your cold?* Mary says: Yes, thank you for asking. I then reply, *I hope everything went smoothly with the repair of your automobile.*

I have worked with people with very minimal sales skills who excelled in this area alone and sold a lot of memberships. This makes our guests feel like we have gone out of our way to make them feel special. We talk to them like a friend and remember the information from our telephone call. Taking simple notes will highly increase your closing percentage and make the perspective member comfortable about purchasing a membership from you. Lastly, we have the outcome. Below are listed the abbreviations that you should use to list the outcome.

For Example:

EN for enroll; **NS** for no show; **MS** for missed sale; **RS** for reschedule; **Pass** for a Pass; **NI** for not interested; and **BB** for if they are going to be back at a later time. **MS**, **RS** and **BB** should have dates for future appointments.

Personal Paycheck Tracking

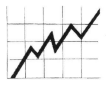

The most important area of the back of the planner is your personal paycheck tracking. This should contain a list of all the memberships you sold for the month as well as prospects' names and telephone numbers, the amount they paid, whether it is an EFT or a prepaid membership, and the commission you received for the sale. You should also have an area for the expiration date of all prepaid memberships, as well as the date they joined. I could not imagine not tracking my personal paycheck, but I still see many salespeople who do not fill out this area of their planner. I would not recommend guessing that the company you work for is going to get your paycheck right every time. If you do not have your exact commission figured out prior to payday, chances are your check will end up in the company's favor. Remember it is against the law for companies not to pay commissions to yoga consultants for the sale of a membership. There are many yoga centers out there that control their bottom line by pulling commission from the consultants. If you work for one of these companies, I would recommend you change your place of employment immediately.

Missed Guests and No Shows

This section in the back of your planner is where you track your missed guest and all of your no shows. This section also has a call-back list to work from as well as a note area to write a message to yourself. This will give you the information needed to cement future appointments. I make a personal goal for myself to get a certain amount of the missed guests back into the yoga center. I even use humor on the telephone if I have called the person several times.

For Example:

"Mr. Thatcher, it is your favorite yoga person on the phone asking if you have stimulated great spiritual and physical growth, which was your original goal, through the perfected art of thinking about it?" "I'm just wondering if you'd like to try a new approach by coming down for a two-week pass at no charge. Is today good or tomorrow better?"

Adding some humor to your job can help, if used correctly.

Business Tacking

Working the business community is a highly effective way of increasing your personal sales. I find it is easy and profitable to trade business products for memberships. These business products can be used for studio give-a-ways, as well as, salespeople and staff enrollment incentives. Business contests, general managers, business owners, and decision-makers influence a large group of people in their company. This is a completely different type of sale; this is a relationship building sale. Most companies do not make fast decisions when it comes to spending money but they will make large decisions financially if the benefit for their company is there. They can also make decisions for placing advertisements, paycheck stuffer, or onsite sales at their place of business. Another benefit is that most of these people will be willing to give you great discounts for their products, since you have gone out of your way to accommodate them.

Renewals

Some yoga centers offer a commission on renewals and some do not. Working renewals is a fast way to make easy money. Most of the time, the member will renew with the first person that reminds them that their membership is coming up for renewal. Be sure to track your renewals in the back of your planner. Also be sure to track any "orphan renewals" that may be falling through the cracks.

For Example:

I am standing at the front desk, checking in the members of our studio, which is what I do at least one-hour every day at different times. I notice that Mr. Johnson's membership is coming up for renewal in six days. I ask Mr. Johnson's if he came in today, because of the huge sale we are having for renewals on yoga memberships. He says, "No, I am here to do yoga today." I respond, "The reason I am asking is because I notice your membership is expiring in six days. Mr. Johnson's, you have come at a perfect time to save money on renewing your membership. And if you are like me, you probably love saving money. Did you want to put one year or two years on your membership? Or would you just prefer to change it to our no hassle monthly plan?"

I list all of my renewals prior to the day of expiration and write down all people who are interested but maybe did not bring their checkbooks or credit cards. Many yoga centers keep the credit card information in their computer, that way you can get an OK for the renewal over the telephone. You would just need a signature when the member comes in next time for a workout.

Lead Box or Contest Box

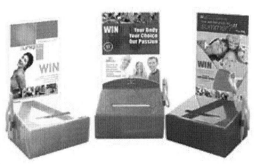

Most sales planners will have an area in the back of their planner for lead box tracking. It will give you an area to track the production of your lead boxes. I do not use the old system of lead boxes, but I still believe in tracking the success of my contest promotions. You can track the success of your promotion, the quality of the leads, and your relationship with the business as well as the dates and times of successful promotions.

Daily planners are a tool that can increase your ability to track all the opportunities that come your way. Opportunities not tracked are opportunities lost. Keeping this information not only shows management that you are paying attention to the details, but that you are willing to exhaust every opportunity and follow up on every lead that is sent your way. If you want to increase your paycheck (and I know you do) keep your mind free. Don't fill it with the little things. Put them in your planner and leave your mind free to do what you have trained to do: close deals.

The sales job is about opportunities. The more opportunities you can have, the more sales you can make! Lost and untracked opportunities are the acts of a fool.

Chapter 6

FRONT DESK SYSTEM

As a member of a team, you will rely on other departments to aid in your success. A team can only be successful if it is willing to use all of the resources available to accomplish a common goal. The first step toward management is the ability to work together to motivate others to do their part and to delegate certain responsibilities. These responsibilities empower your team and your departments. This can help to create a sense of ownership or self-pride. When it comes to front desk systems, a larger responsibility is given to the people who have first contact in most cases with walk-ins, telephone inquiries, check-ins, tracking, and cash register input. If your yoga center is like mine, any guest or member who initially contacts the studio must first go through the front desk process or systems.

Your front desk can have a huge impact on your paycheck.
Don't get on their bad side or you could find that your
paycheck has been manipulated to the lesser.

The front desk personnel should be properly trained and responsible for tracking these valuable guests. They must be deserving of this responsibility. The first area of tracking is member complaints or member issues. We keep a binder for such issues at the front desk. This binder will include member complaints, member check-in issues, broken equipment, or problems in the studio. It may also include suggestions or issues that may be dealt with in our daily production meetings. The front desk may also be responsible for a guest register. A guest register contains all of the information for walk-ins and appointments that come into the studio on a given day. All guests at our studio are given a yoga profile with a tear-off carbon copy on the front. One copy is left at the front desk to be tracked on the guest register and the other one is kept by the yoga counselor for follow up and taking notes. These appointments or walk-ins are tracked and followed up with during our morning production meetings. A pass register will contain a list of all the guests that were on passes and appointment dates for the pass expiration. Front desk systems would also include the first contact with telephone inquiries. These should also be tracked and followed up on in the morning production meeting. Counselors should call up to the front desk and provide the results of all telephone inquiries. It is very important to track all of the guests, passes, telephone inquiries, and appointments that go through our yoga center. The difference between a good studio and a great studio is tracking. This should include tracking advertisements (How the person heard about the studio and not letting one single opportunity fall through the cracks.) Opportunities that are not tracked are opportunities lost. I allocate my Master Appointment Book to my front desk staff. This ensures all yoga counselors are entering their appointments, and the front desk has the ability to greet those appointments using the guest's first name. Remember, your receptionist is the first impression and the last impression you will give to your yoga members, guests, and your staff. This will leave a lasting impression on your company.

Guest Register

Every guest that enters your studio that is interested in a membership should be put on a guest register. A front desk employee should do this. The guest register should also list all the memberships sold for the day. I have found the guest registers offer an accurate closing percentage if used properly. It does not have to be complicated, but it should contain certain information to use for following up with missed guests. I go over this guest register daily in my production meeting to find out what happened to each and every person that came through my studio. This register may prove to be a rich source of information when used properly.

Pass Register

The pass register should have a list of all the guests in your studio that are on passes. This register should have the expiration date of their passes, which should coincide with closeout. Anyone who is given a pass during that month should be in the pass register. These pass holders should be called back during the duration of their pass to find out if they are using the studio. By doing this we show concern to the potential member as well as keep updated for our middle or end of the month party.

TI Register

The TI register is where all of the telephone inquiries (TI) are listed. This register should have the time of the call for an appointment, the source, the name of the caller, and the prospect's work and home telephone numbers. It should also have an area for results. By results I mean whether or not they made an appointment. If yes, for what date and time. If not, what was the reason? Salespeople often forget to update their results immediately after taking a TI. The best way to overcome this problem is to hold the front desk accountable for getting the results or information they could not get from the yoga counselor immediately following the completion of the TI. The manager would then review the TI register daily in the production meeting, highlight the callers that joined, and call back the ones that did not show or were missed sales. Remember, these registers are essential for making sure no calls or potential members are lost or fall through the cracks. Being accountable in these essential areas is crucial to knowing exactly where you or your staff needs improvement.

Chapter 7

MASTER APPOINTMENT BOOK

There are three ways you can operate in a yoga center
1. You can get setup and get prepared.
2. You can wait for walk-ins
3. You can pray!

The master appointment book (MAB) is an important tool used in yoga centers and most service businesses. This important tool is the foundation for team production. If preparation is the key, then this book is the key to success. I believe it would be difficult to fail as a sales manager if you master the art of keeping your MAB filled with quality appointments and follow up on those appointments.

"Yoga is the perfect practice that makes the man perfect."
-Bhagand Geeta

When I use the master appointment book, I make 30 sheets for the whole month and put the names of each yoga counselor on the top of each page. Each separate sheet should have the times and an area next to them for their names and telephone numbers. There should also be an area for the results. The reason we use the MAB is to track all of the leads and sales in the yoga center. Then, through practice and repetition, we learn how to most effectively turn these valuable appointments into revenue. Be sure to track all of your individual appointments for the month, closeouts, and for the next day. You should write your appointments in the master appointment book right when you book them, or call up to the front desk and have them written in for you. Daily goals can also be recorded in this book.

Remember to take notes and get more than one telephone number.

Let's say You take a telephone inquiry. Once you have booked the appointment you call the front desk to let them know. Make sure they write down the telephone number and the appointment date on the TI sheet. Then you write the appointment down in the master appointment book for the time and day that it is scheduled. Include the name, work/home number and cell telephone number if possible. Your planner or personal appointment book should be your master plan for the month. There should be no appointments in any planners that are not also in the master appointment book.

The master appointment book also gives you a list of people to call, such as no-shows, missed sales, and so on. The first job given to a yoga counselor moving into a management role is to manage the master appointment book. The reason for this is obvious. If you can manage the master appointment book; you are managing the first step of production. *The rule for appointments is half show, half join. So if you have 10 appointments a day, 5 will show and 2.5 people will join.* Two point five memberships per day will make you a successful yoga counselor. A good yoga studio manager knows how to run and drive appointments. The master appointment book should be checked several times a day to ensure it is being utilized correctly and consistently. It is a tool that can be used to monitor the progress of the yoga center as well as keep an eye on how the studio is set up for future dates. "Mary, you have no appointments for tomorrow and only two appointments for closeout, and close out is in three days." If you find that you are deficient in a specific area when it comes to appointments, you can have an appointment marathon. For instance, you can have yoga counselors coming into the telephone room for one hour and whoever makes the most appointments in that hour gets a free lunch or a cash bonus. You can have every yoga counselor make one appointment per hour.

For example; coming into the office at exactly twelve o'clock, everyone gets on a telephone and as soon as they book one appointment they are done. You will do that again at one o'clock and again at two o'clock. Each yoga counselor has to have at least four appointments a day. If you have 10 salespeople, that will be 10 guaranteed memberships without a walk-in. If you neglect your master appointment book, your sales and production will be greatly lowered.

Production Meetings

The MAB should be checked in the production meetings for appointments every day, whether or not previous day's goals were hit, in order to set goals for the day. This is the perfect time to do this because during the production meeting all sales counselors should be in attendance as well as have their planners completely filled out. Anything that needs to be added to the MAB can be added at that time.

"Knowing others is intelligence. Knowing yourself is Yoga."
-Lao Tse

Chapter 8

THE STYLES OF YOGA

"Life isn't measured by the number of breaths you take, but the moments that take your breath away."
-Author unknown

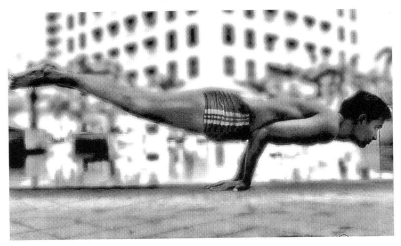

Yoga continues to evolve through the years to meet the needs of every individual from self realization to curing of various ailments. Through the years, Hatha Yoga which is the most popular form of Yoga in the United States and in many parts of the world, continuous to evolve and flourish. Hatha Yoga being the principle branch of Yoga focuses on the physical well-being and believes that the body is the vehicle of the spirit. A lot of different Yoga styles rooted from Hatha Yoga. All these styles seem to balance the mind, the body and the spirit through the Asanas or poses, coordination of breathing and movement of body.

All the Yoga styles seen today have common roots. In fact, the founders of three major styles –Astarga, Iyengar and Viniyoga- were all students of Krishamacharya, a famous teacher at the Yoga Institute at the Mysore palace in India. Two other stules, Integral and Sivananda, were created by disciples of the famous guru Sivananda. No style is better than the other. The style you use is a matter of personal preference or a matter of need.

ANANDA YOGA

Ananda Yoga is a classical style of Hatha Yoga that uses breathing and postures accompanied by silent, positive affirmations to awaken, experience and being to control the subtle energies within oneself, especially the energies of the chakras. Ananda Yoga was developed by Swami Kriyananda, a direct disciple of prahamharsa Yogananda, author of the spiritual classic, "Autobiography of a Yogi."

Ananada Yoga's object is to use those energies to harmonize body, mind and emotions, and above all to attune oneself with higher levels of awareness. So it is a relatively gentle, inward experience and not, an athletic or aerobic practice.

ANUSARA YOGA

Anusara (A-NU-SAR-A) means "following your heart." Anusara Yoga is a powerful Hatha Yoga system that unifies a Tantric Philosophy of Intrinsic Goodness with Universal principle of Alignment. It embodies an uplifting philosophy, epitomized by a "celebration of the heart", that looks for the good in all people and all things.

It was founded by John Friend in 1997, which was mainly influenced by B.K.S Iyenger.

ASHTANGA YOGA

For those who want a serious workout, Astanga yoga may be the perfect Yoga, hence it was often called Power Yoga. Astanga Yoga was developed by Shri K. Pattabhi Jois and is an aerobic, muscleshapping, mind-sculpting, physically demanding workout.

Technique: Participants move through a series of flows, jumping from one posture to another to build strength flexibility and stamina. It also involves performing challenging sequence of poses with Uggayi Breathing and Viniyasas(flow of postures). This yoga style uses a system based on six series of increasing difficulty.

BIKRAM YOGA

It is named after its Founder-Bikram Choudhury who studied Yoga with Bishnu Ghosh, Brother of Paramahamsa Yogananda.

Technique: Bikram Yoga is practiced in a room temperature of up to 100 degrees Fahrenheit, thus be prepared to sweat a lot. Bikram Yoga enthusiasts crank the thermostat to high temperature and then perform a series of 26 Asansa (each held for at least 10 seconds) each of the posture is usually performed twice and also two pranayamas.

Their Yoga sessions start from standing postures, then the Backbends, forward Bends, and Twisting Poses. The postures are accompanied by Kapalabhati Breathing or the "Breath of fire."

Bikram Yoga is designed to "scientifically" warm and stretch muscles, ligaments and tendons in the order of progressive in nature. Practice of this style of Yoga promotes the cleansing of the body, release of toxins and utmost flexibility.

INTEGRAL YOGA

Integral yoga was developed by Swam Satchidananda, the man who introduced chanting to the crowd of the original Woodstock.

Integral Yoga puts equal emphasis on the Pranayama (Breathing Technique), on Meditation and on the Asansa (Physical postures).

Technique: Integral Yoga classes begin with 45 minutes of posture, followed by relaxation, a breathing sequence, and a meditation.

Main Goals of Integral Yoga:

1. Physical Health and Strength
2. Control over all senses
3. Clear, calm and well-disciplined mind
4. Higher level of Intellect
5. Strong and pliable will
6. Love and compassion
7. Pure ego
8. Ultimate peace and joy

IYENGAR YOGA

Iyengar was named after B.K.S.Iyengar. It emphasizes posture and the development of balance and alignment. Iyengar Yoga is one of the most widely practiced yoga techniques in the West and responds to individuals with varying limitations and capacities for accomplishing postures. Iyengar's style is noted for great attention to detail and precise alignment of postures.

Technique:

To support student's explorations of postures, Iyengar yoga make use of a wide variety of props: belts. blocks, pillows and balls. The props helps Iyenga Yogis to achieve the best possible pose, it also provide support and minimizes the risk of getting injured. The yoga poses are held longer and repeated several times, and after attaining mastery of these poses the participants are taught breathing techniques called pranayama.

KALI RAY TRIYOGA

Kali ray Triyoga was founded by Kali Ray.

Technique: This style of Yoga brings posture, breath, and focus together to create dynamic and intuitive flows. These flows combine active and sustained postures following a spinal wavelike movement, economy of motion, and synchronized breath and motion. The flows are systematized by level and can be as gentle or as challenging as desired. Students may progress from basics to advanced as they increase their flexibility, strength, endurance and knowledge of the flows.

There are three stages in Kripalu Yoga:

Stage one: Focuses on learning the postures, proper breathing, and exploring your body's abilities.

Stage two: Involves holding postures for an extended time, developing concentration and awareness of your thoughts and emotions.

Stage three: This stage is called "Meditation in Motion" in which movement form one posture to another arise unconsciously and spontaneously, while the participant is in a meditative state.

Kripalu was named after Swami Kripalvanandayi, a Kundalini Yoga master from India, but was developed by Yogi Amran Desai.

KUDALIN YOGA

Kudalini Yoga was brought to the west by Yogi Bhajan in 1969. This style focuses on the controlled release of the Kundalini (Serpent power) energy which resides at the base of the spine.

Technique: The pratice of Kundalini Yoga involves classic poses, chanting, coordination of breath and movement and meditation. And Kundalini Yoga pays particular attention to chanting and breathing, which aims to get energy moving quickly. Kudalini Yoga rewards Yogis with spiritual transformation and unity consciousness.

SIVANANDA YOGA

Sivananda, one of the world's largest schools of Yoga, is very supportive to beginners. It was developed by Swami. Vishnu-Devananda and named for his teacher Swami Sivananda.

Technique: Sivananda Yoga focuses on the Pranayama, classic

Asanas, and relaxation. It also centers on diet and positive thinking and meditation. Sivananda Yoga practice consist twelve basic Yoga poses that seeks to increase strength, flexibility, proper breathing and meditation.

Sivananda Yoga has over eighty centers worldwide and is considered as one of the largest Yoga schools in the world. "The complete Illustrated Book of Yoga"written by Swami Vishnu Devananda and first published in 1960, was one of the first, and continues to be one of the best, introductions to Yoga available.

JIVAMUKTU YOGA

Jiva, mukti, a Sanskrit word that means "liberation while living", developed by David Life and Sharoa Gannon in 1984. Jivamukti Yoga was developed to promote the educational aspect of the practice and give student access to where these ideas came from. The average Jivamukti student is more educated about the philosophy of Yoga than most Yoga teachers.

Technique: Jivamukti yoga combines a vigorous physical and intellectually stimulating practice leading to spiritual awareness. Each class focuses on a theme, which is supported by Sanskrit chanting, readings, references to scriptural texts, music(from Beatles to Moby), spoken word, Asana and sequencing and Yogic breathing practices. Thus Jivamukti Yoga concentrated on the strong foundation in ancient spiritual traditions of Yoga.

NUDE YOGA

Nude Yoga or naked yoga in its simplest form is the practice of Yoga without wearing any form of clothing. In general, nudist setting is the main difference of Nude Yoga from other styles.

Object of Nude Yoga: To enable you to feel free in your body and to do the poses and exercises without restrictions brought about by Yoga clothes. The important thing about Nude Yoga is its principle. It is doing Yoga poses and exercises with freedom from restrictions of clothing. Understand and accepting this concept can greatly help people in joining a Nude Yoga class without the feeling of discomfort or self-consciousness. Even the practitioners of Nude Yoga think the "universal clothing" is more worthful than the materialistic clothing so they wear the universe as the cloth.

SVAROOPA YOGA

This Yoga style was developed by Rama Berch. Svaroopa Yoga is not an athletic endeavor, but a development of consciousness using the body as a tool.

Technique: Svaroopa Yoga teaches significantly different ways of doing familiar poses, emphasizing the opening of the spine by beginning at the tailbone and progressing through each spinal area in turn. Every pose incorporates principles of Asana, anatomy and Yoga philosophy. It also emphasizes the development of transcendent inner experience, which is called "SVAROOPA" by Patanyali in the Yoga Sutra.

Thus Svaroopa Yoga is a consciousness oriented Yoga that promotes healing and transformation.

VINIYOGA

Viniyoga or what is also known as the "Yoga for wellness" rooted from the principle practiced by Sri. T. Krishnamacharya- that is to develop practices for individual conditions and purposes. His son T.K.V.Desikachar, continued this principle and developed the practice of Viniyoga.

Technique: Viniyoga make use of modified Yoga poses that are designed to meet the specific needs of an individual and to enhance healing, flexibility and strength of joints. Viniyoga poses also intend to promote the feeling of well-being and strength. Practices may also included pranayama, meditation, reflection, study and other classic elements, but the emphasis of Viniyoga practice is on coordinating breath and movement. Key characteristics of the Asana practices are the careful integration on the flow of breath with the movement of the spine and thoughtful sequencing of Asanas. Function is stressed over form.

Chapter 9

THE LANGUAGE

OF SALES

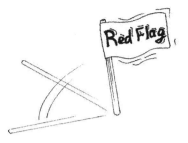

REJECTION WORDS	ACCEPTABLE SUBSTITUTES
Contract	Yoga membership agreement, Paperwork, Form
Cost or Price	Investment or Amount
Down Payment	Initial Investment or Initial Amount
Monthly Payment	Monthly Investment or Monthly Amount
Sell or Sold	Get involved or Get started
Deal	Membership Opportunity
Pay For	Take care of
Sign	Authorize, Approve, Endorse, OK it
Crowded	Popular, Exciting
Sales Person	Yoga counselor, yoga advisor
Dollars	Omit this word altogether—the only possible exception is when the guest is comparison shopping, and your studio is a better value because it will save them so many dollars per month or year
Commission	Fee for service
Objection	Concern
If	When
Cheap	Affordable
Diet	Nutritional Program
Pitch, Spiel.	Presentation
High Pressure	Enthusiasm, Concern
Prizewinner, "up" here	Guest on a free pass or walk-in
Sign up, join.	Get involved, Get started

It is important to know that certain words can create an emotional response from your prospective member. It is important to practice and use only the words that are going to work in your favor.

For Example

"Mom I'm going to the yoga center to get a membership." The mother responds, "Make sure you don't sign anything until you read every thing. Make sure you don't get involved in any contracts!"

People remember these little things. I don't know why but they just seem to pop up when we use certain words. So practice using the right words and your job will be a lot easier, just like second nature.

Chapter 10

HOW TO SPEAK TO A GUEST

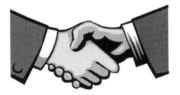 It is amazing how many so-called sales professionals do not understand the basic fundamentals when it comes to speaking to a guest. Rapport building and comfort levels within your perspective member can be established or lost almost immediately. Try to use or remember the things that you learned as a child.

It may sound redundant, but be sure to do the following:

1. Smile. Use a firm handshake. Maintain eye contact.

2. Greetings and introductions. Be sure to introduce yourself and use the guests' name.

3. Building rapport. Be sure to ask questions. Don't give up too much information before you truly understand your guests' intentions. (Use the pre-qualification profile.)

4. Be kind and courteous. Be sure to let your guest do most of the talking. (**You have two ears and one mouth.**)

5. It is important not to be too direct when closing. You must maintain good rapport through five closing attempts. (This will only happen if you use the steps outlined in Chapter 20, How to Overcome Objections.)

Sales language

Only 7 percent of the words that come out of your mouth are communication. It's hard for people to believe that, but it's a fact. Ninety-three percent of your communication has nothing to do with the words that you say; it has to do with your body language, how loudly you speak, eye contact, facial expressions, and your proximity to another person. All of these things come into play when you're communicating with another individual.

One person can talk to a guest or the potential member you are trying to sell a membership to and get absolutely nowhere, and another person can do a full transference of emotions into that guest and sell them a membership by using the exact same words that you just used. The reason why this happens is that you may be talking to your guest, but you are not really communicating with them. You are saying words and those words are coming out of your mouth, but there may be no connection. For example, your facial expressions may be sending a whole different message to your guest.

You can look at someone smile, then laugh and call him or her a name. Or you can scream in someone's face and call him or her a name. These are two vastly different forms of communication. You're saying two completely different things. You have to be aware of how you're communicating. Make a prospect feel that you care. These are techniques that come naturally to some people and are often difficult to teach. It takes a lot of trial and error. Some people have a knack with communication naturally, or they learned it from their parents who were also good communicators. It is important to pin point the communication style of your guest.

The true meaning of sales is the transference of emotions. You will come to the point where you learn how to manipulate through communication. These certain forms of communication are less verbal than you may think. The way we teach sales is we start with teaching you the verbal communication: saying the right words, asking the right questions, getting the person to agree by "using tie downs" all the things that can come across the desk verbally. Through the T.O.

process, and by watching your manager and by listening to other salespeople who may be better than or more experienced than you, you will begin to learn that there are other areas of communication, those which are the non-verbal. This communication is the certain energy that flows across the desk that can't be heard. Have you ever shown a guest the prices, and you see their face turn instantly red, and you start to feel the friction at the table? They haven't said a word, but you can definitely tell. You can see the non-verbal communication. It is coming across the table clear as a bell (the red face and the moving in the seat). You can feel all of the emotions that are coming from your guest. That flow of energy coming across the desk is what I am talking about. A professional knows how to control that energy, harness it, and use it to close more sales.

Why do you get up from a sales presentation? What does that do? Why do we do that? It clears the air. It clears all of those emotions that are flowing back and forth between you and the guest, and it makes them relax. One of your goals is to comfort your guest. Make them loosen up. Make them feel good about making a purchase. They can't do that if they feel the friction across the desk. People project energy. It's as real as anything else. Make sure that you are aware of this. Study this and know that it can hold you back from making sales.

You can say all the right things to a guest and everything may seem to be going good, but there is just something missing. What was missing? They feel uncomfortable and uneasy about buying a membership from *you*. You said all the right things and were nice to the person, but deep down inside the potential member felt that you weren't being honest or they felt that something just wasn't right.

Chapter 11

GREETING AND INTRODUCTION

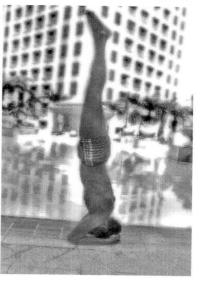

The greeting and introduction is an overlooked but vital aspect of our business. Many sales managers and yoga consultants neglect to devise a uniform greeting strategy when faced with a prospective member.

This is an area that, when focused on correctly, will improve the relationship with the guest, decrease tension, and, ultimately, lead to an increase of sales. There are many different ways of doing this but remember that you never get a second chance to make a first impression. The method I prefer in this situation reads like a script that actors use when memorizing their lines. See the below script for an example.

"How are you?" (Wait for response)

"My name is Mary, and what is your name?" (Wait for response)

"Mr. Prospect, what I would like to do is take a moment of your time to find out exactly what you are looking to accomplish. Then I will take you on a tour of our incredible facility. At that time I will go over all of our different membership options. Sound fair?" (Wait for response)

"Great."

Since I believe in a consistent system approach, I feel it is important to avoid making the introduction too complicated. Many salespeople will not use a system approach for fear it will limit their personality and they are afraid that they may not be able to successfully teach it to new employees. They see it as more of a burden than it is worth, avoiding any type of a standard introduction and presentation altogether. On the contrary, I feel this is the first and most simple area in which to train employees. I make it standard practice to have the yoga consultants rehearse it 50 times before they use it in a real situation. This allows them to become more comfortable with the material, allowing them to become more personable and engaging. Upon completion, I require them to practice it once a month in our production meeting to stay sharp.

One of the most basic fundamentals of building instant rapport can come through the old-fashion art of calling a person by their first name.

Much like the formation of any consistent behavior, practice makes perfect. When consistency has been achieved, improvements and adaptations can be made to instill their own personality into the strategy. A consistent approach and delivery makes for a more relaxed yoga consultant, a more comfortable guest, and, eventually, better results. A relaxed feeling in the guest allows us to defuse many natural reservations buyers have in sales situations, not allowing those reservations to become objections. It is our goal to make the experience more enjoyable for our guest and as easy as possible for ourselves. By eliminating reservations before they become objections, we put the guest at ease and become more efficient at our job.

The goal of a good introduction is to build a strong rapport with our guest. Along with appearance, how we greet them and introduce ourselves is the first critical time to make a good impression. If we do not make a good impression, anything we attempt to do after is much more difficult. By developing a strong introduction and greeting, we build a strong rapport. When a counselor is more at ease with his craft and presentation, his confidence is projected to the guest. It is proven that a more comfortable guest makes for a more satisfied guest, leading you to your ultimate goal. The first opportunity you have to make a prospective member comfortable is during the introduction.

Chapter 12

Building Rapport

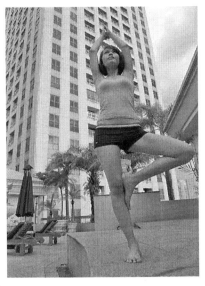

People buy from people they like, and people like people who are like them. What that means is people will most likely feel comfortable around individuals that are in the same economic background as themselves or the same age or even the same nationality. Lets be honest. You don't see high school kids hanging around at the bingo hall or see the janitorial staff at the sales award dinner. It may be a stereotype, but it is also true 99 percent of the time. Are you going to feel comfortable going to lunch with your boss every day when he makes $500,000 a year and the appetizers on the menu are $50 a piece? That would get old pretty fast. Wouldn't you agree? So in order to consistently make sales, you have to build rapport with your guests. You must bring yourself to their level, think how they would think, be patient, and mindful. Maybe this person can't afford to eat at the expensive restaurant every day. People rarely trust those they do not like or feel comfortable with. Be humble and kind. Building a good rapport allows you to build a comfort zone and a trust between yourself and the guest. If there is no trust, there is no sale.

Think of the people you surround yourself with. I am going to go out on a limb and guess that you probably trust and like the people you call your friends. The most successful yoga counselors in this business build mini-relationships with the majority of their guests. A good rapport means that you communicate well with another person, are friendly, and trust one another. This process comes naturally to some people and not so naturally to others, but it is something that you should definitely work on regardless. It sounds complex, but think of each of your clients as a potential friend and you will find yourself more comfortable talking to them. The easiest way to build a strong rapport with your client is by uncovering possible interests that you may have. It is easy for a person to say "no" to a person they do not like, or a person they have nothing in common with. Remember the **K-I-S-S** rule. It means **Keep It Simple Stupid.** Even though you want to build rapport and find common interests, you want to do this in a simple, comfortable fashion. Be careful not to offer too much information about yourself before finding what their interests are. Ask your client questions and find common interests based on their answers. Giving up too much information about yourself before you know the interests of your client can cause problems that are hard to overcome.

For example; Mary is selling a yoga membership to Tom. Tom explains that he is a huge football fan, he lives in the Bay Area, and football is his life. Mary replies, the Bay Area is a beautiful place, and he loves San Francisco. "Go 49ers!" Tom explains that he lives in Oakland, and he is a Raiders fan.

In this situation, the yoga counselor did not find out the proper information before speaking. The yoga counselor was too quick with his response and did not pre-qualify. Therefore, since Tom's life is football, now opposite interests have been established and Mary's sale becomes that much harder. The yoga counselor/client relationship is one of give and take. You will find yourself in situations where you share no common interests with a client. In fact, some of their interests are going to flat-out disagree with yours and may bother you quite a bit. These are the times when you must remember that you are a professional, not a fan, and you are the one who must stay under control. Always try to keep a smile on your face and keep after your goal.

Chapter 13

PRE-QUALIFICATION USING THE GUEST PROFILE

The first thing a lazy yoga counselor may do when taking a short-cut will be to neglect the guest profile. If you are not using the pre-qualification profile, you are missing the boat. Would you go to a doctor's office and have a doctor prescribe medication without knowing your condition? I don't think so. This act would simply be called malpractice! Joining a yoga center is more than simply signing people up on the same membership form one after another. In many cases, you are similar to a doctor prescribing a healthy lifestyle. Such a commitment or this kind of lifestyle change can be difficult. The confrontation of what has caused your guest to seek the help of a yoga center may be elusive.

The only way you may be able to help people make this difficult decision is by consistently finding out what their **NEADS** are, then showing them how you can offer them services, which may work for them in their lifestyle. The letter **N** stands for *now*. You need to know what they are doing now to achieve their yoga goals. The letter **E** stands for *enjoy*. What do they enjoy about what they are currently doing? The letter **A** stands for *alter*. What would they like to alter, change, and improve about their current yoga level? The letter **D** stands for *decision*. Are they ready to make a decision on their own today? And the letter **S** stands for the *solution*. Will you let us, being the yoga professionals, offer you the solution.

Selling Yoga

The first thing people will do when they come into the studio is fill out the Guest Yoga Profile (GYP). The front desk employee will greet them and ask them to fill out the GYP. "It is just a little bit of information to find out exactly how we can meet your needs. It will just take a moment of your time, sound fair?" or "Mary, the reason we ask you to fill out the guest profile is so we can better understand your yoga needs. Since you currently are not a member, it is also an insurance wavier, so you can walk through the studio. It is a requirement to see the facility and it will just take a second to complete, sound fair?" After the guest fills out the profile, a yoga counselor will greet them. The yoga counselor will use the standard introduction we covered in earlier chapters.

It is important to get your guest to sit down. You do that by simply looking into their eyes and sitting down. Do not do it verbally. (It may resemble a command.) It has been proven that most people will not buy things standing up. The yoga counselor will review the front of the profile. It will have an area for their personal information, such as telephone, name, addresses, and how they heard about the studio. How serious they are about exercise? Do they have three hours a week to exercise? Is there any medical reason that would stop them from exercising? Are they are working out now? Have they been a guest before? Is this membership just for them or for someone else also?

After reviewing the front of the profile, you might have some additional questions for the person, especially if they answer the questions on the front in a negative manner. For example, if they say the studio is not convenient, you might want to find out the reason. The key to the GYP is to get deeper answers than just surface answers. It is extremely important to take notes, because your guests will change their answers once they have seen the prices. (If this happens, you can turn over the GYP and show them their original answer.) It may get the guest to open up and tell you what brought them in today. If they say they are just driving by and you just leave them with that, you are not gaining any of the important information. You want to get more in-depth answers.

The second aspect of the GYP is to build rapport and find a common ground. People buy from people they like, and people hang out with people like them. On the back of the profile, you will need to get your guest to open up. When was the last time they were in great shape? How did being in great shape make you feel about yourself? How do the 10 extra pounds make you feel? What are you doing now to hit your yoga goals? Why are these goals important to you? Once they answer these questions, the guest will start to open up a little. You are not going to get an in-depth answer by asking one simple question. They might have a wedding to go to in three weeks. They may have a class reunion coming up. A woman may have seen a picture that made her take action; she may not be unhappy or dissatisfied with her appearance. There are many different things that motivate people to come into a yoga center. Most likely the hot button may not be uncovered by asking only one question. People are not going to tell you, or open up, if you do not mirror and match their energy. They are not going to open up if they think you don't care. They will just sense it. Remember, you are making a first impression here, and this is where you will begin to build rapport and trust. You have to show empathy and understanding. Lastly, people buy from people they like.

You then go through seven or eight questions on the back of profile. You do not want to make it too long, but you do have to ask questions such as, "Do you have three hours a week to exercise?" "Is your family supportive of you joining a studio?" "If the price is affordable, would you like to get started today?" Those questions will help you overcome objections such as "I want to think about it, I want to talk to my wife." "I do not have time." "I do not have the money." That information will be helpful at the end of your price presentation by eliminating or spotting objections early. You might say, "Mr. Prospect, out of the different membership options, which one are you leaning towards?" The potential member might say, "I want to think about it." Then you can come back at them, using the information they provided on the profile and say the following:

"You need to think about it? I can understand how you feel. Other people have felt the same, but what I remember from when we

spoke earlier, you told me you have been thinking about it for a year. So other than thinking about it, is there any other reason to stop you from joining the studio today? If you would not mind me asking, what is it that you are thinking about that you have not thought about it in the past year?"

Then the guest may reply, *"I need to think about the money."* Then you are in the position where you tore down their objection and focus on what their objection really is, money! You can say "Great! Which part is too much, the upfront or monthly?" This is yet another reason why the profile is such an important tool.

The bottom of the profile will have some follow up questions for you to ask. Since everyone who comes to our studio should either join or get a pass, there should be either enrolled or an appointment set to meet with them after the pass has expired. You should have information such as their interests, concerns, or the expiration date of their pass. There should also be an area for follow-up calls. If you have a date on this for the end of their pass, you can file them on the date or the days leading up to that date.

"Mr. Prospect, I just want to call and ask you how the pass is going and to remind you that if you would like to get your pass extended, you can see me tomorrow. I have you down tentatively at three o'clock. If you need to change that, feel free to give me a call."

Using the GYP will take a little more time. The better job you do at filling out this important tool the better your success. As I said early in this book, preparation is the key. The more time you spend pre-qualifying your guests the less time you will have to spend closing them.

Chapter 14

FILLING OUT THE

MEMBERSHIP AGREEMENT

Most salespeople tend to lose their sales right when they begin to fill out the membership agreement. Most of the time, the guest will try to stall by asking questions and hoping to find something in your answer they can use to avoid joining the studio. Some people find it hard to fully agree to a financial agreement. You will see many that agree with everything you say but then will try to find excuses at the end of your presentation in an attempt to find a way out of spending any money. Remember, the K-I-S-S rule, Keep It Simple Stupid. If you give too much information, the guest will find something in your answer that gives them a reason not to join. Always fill out the top of the membership with the personal information yourself. If you give it to the guest, they will stop and hold the pen and start to ask questions. As you fill out the personal information, you want to ask a series of questions that occupy the guest's thoughts. If they are answering your questions, they cannot think of their own questions to ask.

For Example:

   "It is great that you have decided to join the studio today, Mary. Mary, could you spell your last name? And your address? And your telephone number? Mary, did you want to take care of your membership by cash, check, or credit card? And you brought that with you today?"

Simply hold up your hand in the shape of a credit card as you continue to write, and they will almost always reach in and grab their purse or wallet. If they do not reach for their form of payment, ask the same question again, "Have you brought that with you today?"

At that point, you need to get the guest to authorize the membership. You do this by simply explaining the agreement while pointing out each area of the paperwork with your pen. I always put circles or stars next to the area that needs to be signed. I explain, "Mary, this is your membership, we have all of your personal information and you will be getting your card in a moment. Your total investment today is (whatever the total). Your monthly investment I wrote here just to guarantee that your monthly membership is locked in and will not go up. To keep your monthly dues locked in and guaranteed so they will never go up, just go ahead and give me your authorization there." If they hesitate, simply tap your finger on the dotted line and say "right here." If they start to read the agreement, simply tap your finger, and say, "Mary, I will be giving you a copy, and you can read all the rules and details." Again, remember to keep asking questions until all the signatures are finished. "Mary, did you want to make your first training appointment today or would tomorrow be better for you?" The membership agreement should be controlled by the yoga counselor and should never leave your hands. It should be filled out quickly while asking questions. After the guest answers each question, follow immediately with another question.

Overcoming the EFT Objections

Sometimes overcoming the electronic funds transfer (EFT) objections is impossible, but you want to improve as much as possible at overcoming this concern. It is a program that makes monthly dues payments more convenient for the member and for the yoga center. An EFT gives the studio authorization to automatically deduct the amount for the member's dues from either their checking or credit card account. This helps the member by automatically making their payment and keeping their membership active without the concern of making their payment on time. It benefits the studio by having secured access to a check or credit card. This secured billing method is done electronically and uses little time or labor, which will save the studio in the long run. It also shows the company stability to potential investors and/or ownership. When I was new in this business, I was so afraid that the person could sense my own fear of EFTs. Remember, a large percentage of communication is non-verbal. If you are afraid of EFTs, your guest will sense it and will not be willing to use this method of payment. Many people in the past have had bad experiences with electronic fund transfers. Perhaps in your case you may have had such an experience. Remember, in the future, an EFT may be our only way of payment. Computerization is changing everything and most countries outside of the United States only use credit cards and debit cards. All paychecks and bills are sent to your bank or deducted from your bank electronically. Using this system, there is rarely a mistake. I will give you several examples of how to present the easy, no hassle monthly membership program.

Example 1:

"Mary, your membership is taken care of monthly, and your bank will send our bank a check automatically each month, sound fair?"

Example 2:

"Mary, I know you have had problems in the past with automatic withdrawal, but wouldn't you rather save your money and earn interest on it rather than paying your membership in full? The new EFT system at our studio is much more advanced than the old systems. It is the safest and the easiest way for you to take care of your membership. And I can assure you if you have any problems, that you can call me directly, and I will fix it for you immediately. Mary, did you want to pre-pay your membership or do our no-hassle plan?"

Example 3:

"Mary, if you do not mind me asking you a question, what would be the difference between the two payment types? You having an

EFT membership or coming into the studio to pay are the same thing. The only difference is we do not have the ability to hire a large staff to take 10,000 member's checks every month. The only difference for you would be if you did not want to pay for your membership, and you always take care of your bills, right Mary?"

Example 4:

Mary says, *"I do not want anyone to have access to my account."* I respond, "Mary, the only one who has access to your account is your bank, and you are authorizing your bank to send our bank $25 per month. We have no access to your bank. Any mistake that would be made would be made by your bank and would be your bank's responsibility. Take a look at the agreement, Mary. It shows that you are authorizing only $25 dollars a month on the first of each month and nothing more."

Example 5:

Mary says, *"I do not do anything automatically out of my account."* I respond, "Mary, I do not do anything automatically out of my account either. But I think you would agree with me that the fees for my checking account are taken out automatically by my bank. Fees for bounced checks or overdraft charges, new check charges, or annual fees are taken out automatically. So I think we can both agree that the future is going to only leave room for this form of payment. Most companies are even deducting taxes automatically from our directly deposited paychecks. So I think you would agree that in most cases, this is our only option."

Remember that an EFT membership is more convenient for the client, the studio, and you. What you as the professional must communicate to the client is that this form of payment exists for their convenience. Like anything else, if they see how the program benefits them and they trust what you say, they will be more likely to agree to it.

Chapter 15

MIRRORING AND MATCHING

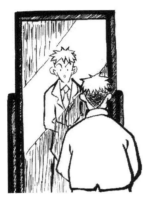

Remember, people buy from people they like, and people like people who are like them. It is important to adjust style and personality to be in touch with your guest. What does this mean? It means having the ability to change the way you act, talk, and the speed in which you react or walk, everything you do to set your rhythm in synch with the person that you are with. This is not something that I can outline for you. It is not something that is easy to teach. But this is an effective tool.

For Example:

If you have a person who is shy, you cannot be aggressive. If you have a person who walks slowly, you cannot walk fast.

This area of your arsenal can go much deeper. You have to be like a chameleon, which is a lizard that can change its color and shape to meet its surroundings.

For Example:

If you have a 60-year-old woman, it will be hard for you to understand how she feels if you are 25. In this case, your best chance of making her feel comfortable is if you can make her feel like she is buying a membership from her 25-year-old grandchild. Tell her how you have a grandmother and how much you love her. You can even make a comment such as, *"We have lots of people your age practicing yoga in our studio,"* and maybe something sly such as, *"She would probably fit in great with the rest of the 29-year-olds."* Learning to mirror and match takes time, and it takes experience.

Watch the other salespeople that have been around for a while. I must say that my success in managing yoga centers has come from my ability to match up the right yoga counselor with the right guest. The studio I am currently managing has a large sales staff. They have all different kinds of personalities. They are different ages and come from different ethnic backgrounds. If our guest is shy, I give the guest to our shyest counselor. If the guest is young, I give him or her to our youngest counselor. If the guest speaks Spanish, I give him or her to our counselor that speaks Spanish. If the guest is a female, I give her to a female. This matching up of the right counselors with the right guests has highly increased our closing percentages. Could you imagine if your studio just went on a regular rotation, and young kids were matched up with the old men, and the person that spoke Spanish ends up with the person who does not speak Spanish? Believe it or not, there are still managers not involved in this important aspect of the business. Reading the newspaper in the back office and not taking advantage of matching up personality types will reduce your paycheck.

Chapter 16

YOGA & ITS POPULARITY

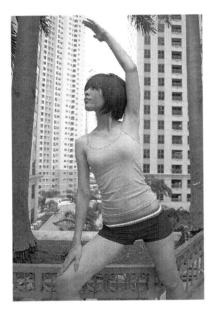

Yoga, the ancient practice of postures, breathing and meditation, is gaining a lot of attention from the material world that its serious practitioners are trying to develop. The soaring popularity of Yoga that has originated in India is becoming the most popular physical and mental practice of choice for thousands of urbanites across the world.

Yoga is already widely practiced in such countries as the United States and Australia. In most Asian cities, over the past many years Yoga has become one of the most popular forms of exercise and, in some cases, a very profitable business. A glance through recent issues of the monthly yoga journals clearly illustrates the focal point that Yoga is becoming a big business, with an estimated regional turnover well in excess of $500 million.

Americans spend some 2.95 billion dollars a year on Yoga classes, equipment, clothing, holidays, videos and more. Studies have found that roughly 16.5 million people were practicing Yoga in the United States early last year, in studios, gyms or at home, up 43% from 2002.

Flooding The Market

Established sellers of Yoga gear such as Hugger Mugges and Gaiam have been flooded with competition in the market for Yoga mats, incense, clothing and fancy accoutrements ranging from designer Yoga bags to eye pillows.

Vancouver British Columbia based Lululemon Athletica, for one, has seen sales of its Yoga apparel rise to $100 million since Canadian entrepreneur Chip Wilson founded the company in 1998.

A lot of investors are being attracted to the trend of Yoga, one of the most popular Highland Capital partners has nearly 14 locations in Southern California and New York.

Corporate types have indeed latched on. Rob Wrubel and George Lichter, best known as the men behind the Internet site Ask Jeeves, in 2003 provided refinancing for Yoga Works, which was founded in the late 1980's. Another expanding business, Exhale, markets itself as a "Mind Body Spa", with tony locations in Los Angeles, New York and other Urban Areas that combine Yoga classes with facials, massage and alternative treatments such as acupuncture.

It's about beauty and ascetics, not about opulence, that's how it has entered into the Mind Body Spa of Hollywood and Original Power Yoga was practiced by Madonna, Sting, Woody Harrelson, William Dafoe and more. Western people have become attracted to the practice of Yoga and they have followed their role models.

In some markets there is a scarcity of information on the number of people practicing. This is probably due to the relative novelty of the phenomenon and the variety of establishments offering Yoga classes.

Popularity of Yoga in Singapore, Hong Kong

If you live in Hong-Kong, Singapore or Taipei, it is difficult to count the number of Yoga studios that are already existing. But it is estimated that at least one yoga studio is initiated per week.

News paper and magazines run yoga-studio ads on a daily basis. Advertisements are also developed on the basis of yoga themes for other products. Yoga classes are offered at gyms, beauty salons, clubs and community centers.

In Hong Kong though, there are more than 60 studios, and Pure Yoga, the largest chain, has an estimated 18,000 members across their locations. In Singapore, the practice of yoga has surged in the past few years almost to a national craze. According to a survey of the Singapore Sport Council last year, an estimated 55,000 people practiced at least once a week – a large number in a country of only 4 million people.

REASONS

A large number of beginners, especially females are attracted to the yoga studios in order to lose weight. That also explains the growing popularity of the so-called "HOT" Yoga styles.

Many like practicing yoga because is a way to build strength and at the same time, to increase flexibility. There is also a growing number of physicians recommending Yoga to their patients for a variety of conditions, from high blood pressure to back pain.

Patrick Wee, the founder of True Yoga, a company that owns five studios in Singapore, Bangkok, Taiwan and Kuala Lumpur, believes that the growing popularity of yoga is also due to the growing need to pursue a healthier life style.

Perhaps a less obvious reason for the popularity of Yoga in Asia is that this ancient tradition is especially effective in creating a sense of peace and relaxation, primarily to balance out stressful lifestyles in modern Asian societies and to complement the search for inner peace.

Another reason is the pollution that has become a plague in most Asian cities. In such an environment, outdoor exercise is not much of an option. Yoga provides a good indoor alternative that can be practiced virtually any time of the year.

There is no question that a new breed of Yoga schools has also contributed to the growing popularity of this practice. No longer small one-room schools tucked away in some bohemian part of town, the new temples of yoga are the mega-studios. These are in prime shopping or office locations and sprawled over 1,400-1,800 square meters, designed more with an eye for the luxury tropical resort than for the fitness club.

Yoga has gained its popularity more for its physical, physiological, and spiritual benefits. The practice of yoga relaxes the entire body and gives us a healing sense of peace, so that the physical benefits have gained popularity in professional athletes, as the breathing practice rightly called "Pranayama" increases lung power for athletes, and avoids diseases caused by respiratory problems.

The major reason for the popularity of Yoga is the simplicity in practicing it; it does not require costly clothing, costumes, larger places and it can be practiced anytime, anywhere under guidance.

The concentration and meditation technique teaches us to balance mood, to cope with stressful situations, pain management, quiet our chattering minds, slow our thoughts and discover connection and how to open to your light inside and out. The relaxation techniques of Yoga teaches us anger management and helps our physiological mechanisms to be regulated. It bring the healing light to our bodies to help with illness and to learn to channel energy and to open up to the healing energy around us, in our bodies, hearts, minds and souls. For these spiritual energy benefits Yoga is widely accepted in China and Japan.

Recently there is the surge in the popularity of Yoga is because Yoga also has curative properties. On understanding this in India many schools and universities started to conduct research on the-medical aspects of Yoga. Yoga has been found to cure almost 75% of the disorders. Regular practice of Yoga increases the immunity power in the body which helps in preventing diseases from entering the body. Thus Yoga augments the principle of "Prevention is better than a Cure."

The reason that Yoga has gained more ascendancy in Asia is because its principles coincide with the traditional philosophy of Zen Buddhism and Tibetan Buddhism, As most all Asian people want to return somewhat to the older traditions from the modern lifestyle, they choose Yoga and meditation tas the best path way for them.

On understanding the physical, physiological and spiritual benefits of Yoga, many corporate companies have indeed latched on to this ancient tradition, science and art within culture, religion and world view to transport them to the other side of the world. Thus Yoga has gained the popularity in the recent years for its principle aim to have a peaceful mind and eternal life.

Chapter 17

UNIFORMS AND NEATNESS

Would you go on a date with a girl who dresses trashy? Would you show up to your wedding wearing shorts and sandals? Probably not. In life, you will never get a second chance to make a first impression. The same goes for the business world. You want to increase your percentage in every way possible and dressing properly for this situation is one way of accomplishing that. People stereotype. If you want to be a professional, you have to look professional. If you want your staff to respect you, you will have to look professional. There is an old saying: "If you want to be better than 75 percent of the staff, all you need to do is show up to work every day. If you want to be better than 80 percent of the staff, then you need to show up to work, on time every day as scheduled. If you want to be better than 90 percent of the staff, all you need to do is to show up to work on time as scheduled dressed in a uniform. If you want to be better than 99 percent of the staff, all you need to do is to show up to work, on time, with a uniform, and have a plan.

The appropriate uniform in this business is either business attire or a yoga sweat suit. The uniform should match the rest of the staff. You should have clean shoes, your shirts should be ironed, and you should have a white or black T-shirt underneath. (Avoid black uniforms as bad guys in movies wear black.) There should be nothing special on your uniform that would differ from your staff. You should also wear a nametag with your title, because people feel more comfortable when they can call you by your name. If an improper uniform costs you to lose one sale, it is not worth it. If your haircut offends one person, it is not worth it. People may see your tattoo and be afraid to give you their credit card, because they associate tattoos with crime. Conservative is the best.

Remember, this is your job and your livelihood so if there is an adjustment to be made, suck it up and make the change while you are at work. The styles of today are not professional looking or conducive to a business situation. Comb your hair, maintain facial hair, cover tattoos, take earrings out of the nose and eyebrow, wear clean clothes, and get the job done. If you neglect these areas, it will not make you a bad person but it will cost you in the number of sales. Why do you think the president of the United States wears the same blue-striped tie and plain suit all of the time? It is because he does not want to offend a single person. Your job may not be as important as the president's, but the fact remains if you want to be taken seriously you have to dress for the occasion.

Chapter 18

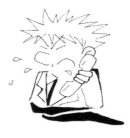

HOW TO DEAL WITH A TOUGH CUSTOMER

With the increasing number of yoga centers, we are noticing that it has become more difficult to deal with the consumer. They are more educated and often times put up resistance to a sales situation right away. It seems as though some days you cannot encourage a single guest to complete the yoga profile, or even stop long enough to see the membership options. Remember, no matter how good you are, you are not going to make every sale or close every telephone inquiry. It is important to improve your percentages as much as possible. So here are some pointers and different techniques that have worked for me when dealing with these types of clients.

You want to try and match your guest's energy. If they are speaking loud, you speak loud. If they are walking fast, you walk fast. If they are not letting you talk, do not listen to them talk. If they act like they are not interested in joining the studio, then you act like you are not interested in signing them up. These steps may not be the most politically correct, but they definitely work. I can get almost every tough customer to settle and sit down, avoid complaints, or fix the problems they may have. I truly feel that customer service in a yoga center is a little bit different. There is a time when our members just want to vent, and there are other times they just want to be heard out. If you apologize to every member in your studio when they have a complaint, you will lose control of your studio and your members will make all the rules. Remember, these people are in your studio every day. It is different than a restaurant or a grocery store.

For Example:

A guest walks into the studio and says, *"I do not want any sales pressure. I do not want a tour. I am not filling anything out. I want the price sheet, now!"* In the exact same manner, same voice, same proximity, same tone, I would say, *"My name is Ron, and what is your name? Welcome to the studio. Since you are not interested in seeing our studio, and you are not interested in helping us understand your goals, I would imagine you are just here to sign up today."* The guest says, *"No. I just want prices!"* I respond by saying, *"Unfortunately, you misunderstand our business. I wish that every person was the same, and every person had the same goals, but this is not the case. And for me to design a membership option for you in 20 seconds would not be fair. Would you go into the doctor's office and say 'give me medicine!' Of course not. The doctor will lose his job for malpractice. I take my job as a yoga professional very seriously. I have helped thousands of people change their lives. I would suggest you go into a studio where they are interested in signing people up and making money, and not to a studio like ours, where we are interested in helping people get results."*

Tough customers exist in every business. People that scream and yell do it because it works for them. The more and more customer service people apologize, the more the member will yell. The true yoga professional will simply tell the member that they are the only one that can help them fix the problem. If they cannot be adult enough to lower their voice and not swear, the problem will never be fixed and will continue forever. Or we can sit down like adults and solve the problem right now. I do not care how good a yoga counselor you are; you will never make every person happy. There are people in the world that will create problems in every situation. They intentionally cause controversy. It is a way of life, and it makes them feel good to make your life miserable. In a yoga center, you do not have to feed into this game.

Never deal with problems or complaints at the front desk. Take the problem to an office right away!

Chapter 19

THE TOUR

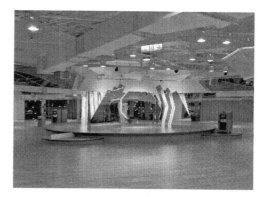

There are many different tours used by many different salespeople. I believe that sales is a process that involves asking questions to make people think for themselves and make decisions for themselves. On the tour, I use more statements than I do in any other areas because you do need to tell the guest what is in the studio and what the studio can do for them. I use a three-step process in order to let the guest realize that they may not know as much about yoga as they think they do. Remember, if they were getting the results on their own that they would not be coming to a yoga center. Telling is not selling and by telling your guest that they are out of shape or that they need to focus on a certain aspect only instills doubt in their minds. On the other hand, if you can get them to admit or say it, then in their mind it is true. I prefer to start my tour in the area that is of the most interest to the guest. I do this for a simple reason. You can lose the guest's attention during the tour if all they are thinking about is the yoga program. If you show them the yoga program first, that question will be out of their mind and they will be more open to understanding the rest of the facilities. I then use my three-step system to let them decide for themselves if they think they need the help of our instructors and our yoga center.

Step 1: A statement of fact: *"We have 50 treadmills. The treadmills are used for cardiovascular and respiratory conditioning. They are state of the art and have springboards to protect your joints from injury."*

Step 2: I then ask two to three questions that will make the guest understand that we have information that can help them be more successful and accomplish their goals faster than they would working out on their own. *"Mary, do you know what your target heart rate is?" "Mary, are you aware of the exact time, intensity, and duration that you should do cardio exercise to achieve optimal results?"*

Step 3: Step three is a tie down. A tie down is a question that invokes a "yes" response or gains agreement from the client. To help me accomplish this, I simply nod my head when I use a tie down. *"Mary, it sounds like you may benefit from having one of our certified professionals tell you about target heart rate."*

I use this three-step system in several areas of my studio. It would be difficult for a guest to not know the answers to all of these questions and still say they do not need any help. Also remember that some small talk and rapport building is important on the tour. You do not want to sound like you know it all. I listed some questions that you can ask and the areas in which you can ask them, as well as some great tie downs to make your tours more effective. There are many ways to give a tour, and this is just one of them. It gives you the room to add your own style, and you should try to create excitement and awe wherever possible.

Proper Food Intake

Questions

1. How important would you guess that proper food intake is for you to accomplish your yoga goals?

2. How is your food intake right now?

3. Did you know that "hunger" is actually the biggest enemy to accomplishing body fat reduction?

Tie Downs

1. Proper food intake is actually 60 to 70 percent of your success, so can you see the importance of meeting with

Tom to have a meal plan strategy customized according to your lifestyle and food preferences, correct?

2. Can you see how meeting with Tom will eliminate all of your guesswork related to food intake and accomplishing your goals? That is something you are definitely interested in, right?

Proper Cardiovascular Prescription

Questions

1. Are you aware of what your target heart rate is? Do you know why it is important?

2. Are you familiar with the Frequency, Intensity, Time, and Type (FITT) principle?

Tie Downs

1. How would you like to have an instructor show you the least amount of cardio necessary to accomplish your goals?

2. Isn't it nice that we have instructors to eliminate your guesswork and design the most effective program for you?

Proper Supplementation

Questions

1. Did you know that if you are exercising and you are not supplementing, your metabolism is probably not functioning optimally?

2. Did you know that it is well documented that if you were to get all of the nutrients your body needs to truly be functioning at its best from food alone that you would have to eat more than 2,500 calories a day? How close do you think you would get to your goal of eating 2,500 calories a day?

Tie Downs

1. There are a lot of products here that do a lot of different things. Fortunately you do not need to take all of them, right? And even more fortunate, isn't it nice to have a yoga professional that will educate you so you do not have to figure it out all by yourself?

2. Aren't you glad that you can work with a yoga professional to eliminate all of your guesswork when it comes to supplementation?

Proper Resistance Training

Questions

1. Are you aware of why resistance training is important for someone with your goals of reducing body fat?

2. What have you done for resistance training in the past? Do you feel like what you have done got you the best possible results?

Tie Downs

1. How would you like to work with a instructor and get set up with the ideal number of sets, reps, and rest periods, and which exercises are best for achieving your goals?

2. Does it make sense that if you are going to be ultimately set up for success you would want to have a certified instructor customize your program?

Swimming/Jacuzzi/Sauna

Questions

1. What has been your experience with swimming?

2. Do you know what type of results you will receive from swimming?

3. How often do you swim?

4. Do you have any friends that are interested in swimming?

Tie Downs

1. Do you prefer to relax in the Jacuzzi or the sauna?

2. How would you like to have your instructor build swimming into your cardio routine in order to achieve your goals?

3. Can you see yourself coming in for a relaxing swim, sauna, or Jacuzzi?

4. Isn't it nice to come in to the wet area and relax after a stressful day?

5. Do you think you will be using the wet area every time you come in or will it just be using it occasionally?

Again, these are just suggestions. You are free to include some questions of your own. These questions and tie downs have been tried and tested for many years and have been met with outstanding results.

Chapter 20

THE COMMITMENT QUESTION

Avoid giving too much information. Only give information once you have some commitment from your guest.

The commitment question is a simple question that you can use as a new yoga counselor to help you overcome objections. Once you have been a yoga counselor for a while, you probably will not have to ask this question. When you first start selling, the question helps you gain commitment from the guest. The reason we ask a direct commitment question is for a simple reason. To the guest, the knowledge about costs will solve all their yoga needs. But once they know the price, they will be satisfied and give you excuses so they can leave; there is no reason for them to join the studio once that information is gained. When they have the price, they have everything they need. People want things more when they cannot get them or they cannot have them.

The yoga center business started just like every other business. The guest would be given the price sheet and then, unlike other businesses, the guest would never come back. So, yoga centers started to evolve and understand that our business was different. We had to bring in and train professional salespeople to help stop the procrastination process. The consumer had to be treated more like an addict rather than a shopper or consumer. Think of your guest as a poor lifestyle addict in need of your help. We do not want to beg them or tell them to join the studio. We ask the guest to help us help them. Instead, we avoid giving them too much information, forcing them to give us a commitment in exchange for the information they desire. The question I ask is, *"If I can give you a good price, would you want to get started today?"* If the person says, *"No,"* you ask, *"Even if I can give you a very good price, would you not want to join the studio today?"* If the person says no, then you ask, *"What if the membership was $20 for the whole year?"* If they say, *"There is no way for you to do that price."* You can say, *"No. I can do it for free, but I am not going to!"* If they say they will join if the price is $20, then you say, *"So it's just the money."*

Once you get that question out of the way, you can break down their every objection. That way, if they say later, *"I want to think about it,"* you can say, *"You just said that if I could get you a good price, you would join the studio today, so how much is too much?"* Do not give an accurate membership cost without them answering the commitment question with a yes.

I know this sounds strange, but I will get every guest to commit to joining if the price is right. If they say no to that question before they walk back to the table, you can simply walk them out of the studio quickly, shake their hand, and say, *"Come back when you are ready to join. Yesterday we had a great sale. Unfortunately that sale is over, and our new pricing has not come in yet. If we sit down and go over different membership options, it would be a waste of your time. Later on today, we will have all new membership prices. You will not be able to qualify for the special that I offered to you earlier. I do not want to waste both of our time by offering you yesterday's pricing."* Almost instinctively, they will ask, *"What was the price?"* You have now made them commit to asking you a question and are in control of the information that they need. You can then reply, *"That is not going to matter, because you cannot get that price when you come back. The sale is only for today."*

People do not want things that are too easy to get. I know this sounds like it is not the best move from a customer service stand point but remember, Our job is to help people stop procrastinating and get started. If we need to accomplish that by using odd methods or by being up front and honest with the possibility of sounding rude, that is what we need to do. We will not be able to help very many people accomplish their goals by giving them all the information, handing them a price sheet, and saying go home and think about it. If you do, the guest will lose their interest and the motivation it took for them to come into the studio. You will never see many of those people again, and you will not have done your job.

Chapter 21

PRICE PRESENTATION

The price presentation should be brief. It should quickly cover what each membership includes or involves. I have found that if the price presentation is done poorly, it will not completely kill your membership sale, but it will make it more difficult. There are several different ways of presenting membership options. If the prospect asks you what the processing fee is for, you can simply say, *"This is what our company pays to have your membership processed. It includes putting you in the computer, getting you a membership card, the cost of your orientation instructor"* Make sure that all of the questions are out of the way before showing price. Try to ensure that your guest is committed to join the studio today if you can find them the right price. Here is the price presentation that I have used for many years.

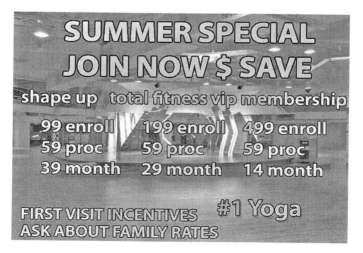

For Example:

"Mary, we have three membership options to choose from. The first one is great, and it is called our *Shape Up* program. You only pay a little bit upfront to get started, but a little more on the monthly investment. The initial amount is a one-time investment to get you started. The second membership option is our *Total Fitness* program. It is a little more to get started, but it has a lower monthly investment. For the last package, there is quite a bit more upfront to get started, but it has the best monthly rate. You are actually buying your dues down, and as you can see, it has the lowest monthly investment and makes the most sense in the long run. It also comes with extra services such as advanced one on one classes, a VIP locker, laundry service, and parking. As you can see, this membership is obviously the best value for you in the long run. Now, all these packages are great and will help you to accomplish all of your goals in our studio. I will stand behind you in any decision that you make today. Out of the different membership options, which one are you leaning toward?" As the guest points to one membership, you simply hold out your hand (preparing to shake it) and say, "Welcome to the studio."

Remember to assume that the guest is just going to join the studio. Just assume you have closed the deal and immediately start filling out the membership agreement. Start by asking questions so they cannot bring up objections or stall. Remember, they cannot think of questions or objections if they are busy answering your questions. The person asking the questions is controlling the conversation. If they bring up an objection, show empathy, isolate, overcome, and get the objection broken down to the money. Remember to remain calm, even if you feel that the person is giving you a large amount of money. If you have anxiety, your guest will sense it. Also note that a lot of people have plenty of money. What may seem like a lot of money to you may be peanuts to somebody else. If the person tries to act silly as you are starting to fill out the membership agreement, that means they are trying to change the subject or are trying to stall. They are asking you questions so they can find something in the answer that will allow them to stall or not join. Answer all of those questions with questions of your own. *"How many yoga classes do you have?" "What yoga classes are you looking for?" "What time does the studio open?" "What time will you be using the studio most?" "How much is it if I want to bring a friend?" "Did you want to put your friend on the VIP guest list?"* That is the price presentation, and it is simple. You ask the commitment question, and then you ask them if they have any additional questions. At that point you can go over the different membership options.

Chapter 22

HOW TO OVERCOME OBJECTIONS

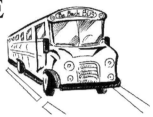

The seven most common objections will be the weaponry used by your guests to stop you from enrolling them. These procrastination techniques have been used successfully for years. The sooner you learn to overcome them, the sooner you will start to help people improve their lives.

- Spouse (I want to talk husband or wife. Mom or dad.)
- Shop around (I want to go see other studios.)
- Time (I don't have it.)
- Try it out (I want to use my pass first. I will join after my workout.)
- Think about it (I will be back.)
- Group/Friends
- Too expensive

How long will you wait to learn how to overcome this weaponry? This will get used against you on a daily basis. The faster you feel comfortable hearing the excuses and overcoming them, the better yoga counselor you will become. **Drill, drill, drill.**

How to Handle Objections

1. Hear them out. If you cannot hear the problem, you will not be able to understand their concerns.

2. Feed it in back a form of question. "You want to think about it"?

3. Show empathy. "You want to think about it? I can understand you want to think about it. This is a big decision. Other people have been thinking the same way."

Remember Three Key Words:

1. **Feel**: "I can understand the way you feel."

2. **Felt**: "Other people have felt the same way."

3. **Found**: "But we have found out that once you have started your membership, it is going to the best decision you have ever made.

Isolate: "Other than thinking about it, is there anything else preventing you from joining the studio today?"

Overcome: "If the price was only $20 for the whole year would you still want to think about it? "No? So it is just the money."

Get it down to money. We cannot control what their husband is going to say, the distance they live, or whether or not they have time. But we can change the price. We can work with different membership options to fit their needs. The other way to overcome this is by changing the subject. Keeping the subject on the money when they want to change it to something else.

"Do you want to think about it? The up-front or the monthly?"

"Maggie, you want to talk to your husband? Do you want to talk to him about the upfront or the monthly?"

Most objections will center around money. Money is a delicate issue in which to deal, so people will avoid talking about it and find other excuses to dwell on. You have seen the excuses above and probably relied on a few yourselves from time to time. Objections are common in this business, and you have to learn to overcome them if you are going to be successful.

Chapter 21

CLOSING

I feel that most salespeople would agree that the bottom line in sales is closing the deal. If everything goes great, you do everything perfect, and you do not close the sale, nothing else matters. Nothing was really accomplished, and no money was made. On the other hand, if you do everything wrong, and you close every sale, then from a financial and business standpoint, you are successful. That is why people who are closers are held in such high regard in our business today. We can compare this to the quarterback who comes in and throws the touchdown pass in the final seconds to win the game or to the pitcher who comes in to closeout the inning. The people who can get it done are the ones who make big money. No matter how you get there, the end result is to win. This is the reason there is such competition and why so many people in our business, or who are successful in this business, are ex-athletes who have thrived and excelled when faced with competition.

There are seven steps used by top producers. These are the areas that when focused on will make the difference between closing every sale and missing every sale. This information is the Holy Grail of our business. If you follow the advice, you will see a marked improvement in the area of closing. Although I can offer you ideas on what to say, what you say is not half as important as what you do and how you say it. I have taken over a million sales, and one of the common things I hear from the new salespeople is, and I quote, *"You just said the exact same thing I said, and they would not join with me. But they joined with you!"* I always reply, *"Although we said the same words, you and I communicated something totally different."*

Remember to practice these seven steps. Reading them will do nothing for you. We do not sell memberships to books; these must be practiced in role-playing situations. Think of it like a football player who studies the playbook. He must know the playbooks forward and backwards to be successful. But simply knowing the playbook is not enough. He needs to put that knowledge to work during practice and games in order to perfect his craft. He must learn to overcome, improvise, and adapt to many different situations as they happen. You are the quarterback of your career. I will provide the playbook, but you must provide the hard work and dedication it takes to perfect it for you to be successful.

The Seven Steps to Closing

1. Close too often and too early rather than too seldom and too late.

2. You must be assumptive. (always assume the sale!)

3. Mirror and match, people feel comfortable with people like them.

4. Use the force, 93 percent of communication is non-verbal.

5. Control the conversation with questions. Answer questions with questions.

6. You must overcome five objections. Most sales in the world are made only after the fifth closing attempt.

7. Do not be afraid of silence. After asking any question, be quiet–the first one to talk loses the battle.

Close too often and too early rather than too seldom and too late!

You want to close too often and too soon rather than too seldom and too late. You do not want to let the opportunity to close a sale pass you by. Closing too soon rather than too late allows you to get a peek at the person's intentions or to gage their interest level. I always say, relatively early in the close, "Which one of these different membership options are you leaning towards?" The potential member will tell you which membership he or she is considering, and I quickly say "Welcome to the studio!" It is quick and assumptive, but you may just find the person thanking you and going along with it. If it does not work, the guest will usually let you know. It is a gamble worth taking because usually the member will take it as lighthearted and fun and not become too upset. Even if this does happen, you have succeeded in establishing a relaxed situation by making the person laugh. Either way, you are closer to your goal. Here are a couple more examples of questions you can ask to try and close early:

"Were you going to come to your first work out dressed and ready to go? Or were you going to need a locker and a towel?"

I see rookie sales counselors making the following mistake all of the time. "Out of these three membership options, which one are you leaning toward?" The potential member says he likes the VIP membership. The common mistake that a rookie counselor makes is that they will then ask, "Is the upfront too much or is it the monthly that you are more concerned with?" They have over-anticipated an objection before the client provided one. *Do not do this!* Do not put potentially harmful words to your sale in the person's mouth. The potential member just said they were ready to buy the membership, so do not give them the option to now say it is too much. When faced with this situation, all is not lost. You can still overcome and meet your objection, but you have made it harder on yourself.

The magic "yes" is not going to fall out of the sky. It just does not happen this way. Very rarely does the person say, "I'll take that membership." What you want to do is gain their agreement along the way with questions so they are no longer saying no. If they are not saying no, they must mean yes. Assume the sale; you can never close too early.

You must be assumptive!

Being assumptive is probably the best close in sales. Just having an assumptive attitude and saying, "Great, welcome to the studio," makes the guest think that it is what everybody does and will simply figure this must be how it works. A lot of the time what we do as yoga professionals is offer the prospect an opportunity to haggle by not closing the deal right away while we have the opportunity.

I used to work for a talented Individual whose favorite close was to show the prospect the different membership options and say, "You know what? I think this one is best for you." Then he would start filling out the agreement. As soon as the guest started to talk, he would ask them a question. "Did you want to pay cash or credit card, your first name, last name, address?" and so on. It was so assumptive that he did not even give the person a chance to think it over. He would just start writing. Many times that closing technique worked. But it takes a lot of time to get to that level unless you are just a natural yoga counselor.

Use the force!

Use the force to close the sale. You may think this sounds ridiculous as a new yoga counselor but, hey, it worked for Yoda. You may think that selling is just pressuring people and talking them into doing something they do not want to do. Actually, sales has little to do with the words that come from your mouth. Think about this: If you were to go in a dark room with another person, is it or is it not a fact that that a person gives off heat? Is it or is it not a fact that that person gives off energy? Is it or is it not a fact that that person makes sounds when breathing or moving? You can smell them. With no sight and no words, there are many other forces that can affect communication. Within words, there are certainly many forces. You can insult someone with a smile and it seems like a joke; joke around with him or her with a frown, and it seems like an insult. Only 5 to 10 percent of the words you say are communicated by just the words you speak.

Here are some of the other factors:

1. The tone of your voice.
2. The speed in which you talk.
3. The proximity between you and your guest.
4. How loud you are.
5. Fear in your voice.
6. Your facial expressions. (Many salespeople blush or make faces, and they are not aware they are doing it!)
7. Eye contact.
8. Ability to remain calm.
9. The speed in which you ask or answer questions.
10. The clarity of your voice.
11. Respect level.
12. Using slang.

I think you get the point. I could go on, but I think you are a newfound believer in the force. As I watch my sales area from 30 feet away, unable to hear any verbal communications, I am aware of what is taking place at each and every table. My Yoga professionals will often ask me, "How did you know what was going on?" I simply say, "I do not have to hear what you are saying, I can see everything you are saying just fine."

Mirroring and Matching!

I covered this chapter earlier in the book. It is important to mirror and match at all times with your guests.

Lead with Questions!

The person asking the questions is the one in control of the conversation. When it comes down to closing a sale, your guest will ask a lot of questions that they do not really care about hearing the answers to. These are stalling tactics. They are looking for something within your answer that would give them a way out. For instance, you are filling out the paperwork, and Mary asks, "Who teaches your step class?" An inexperienced yoga counselor might answer, "Oh, it is Jonathan, he is one of our best instructors." Mary says, "I do not feel comfortable doing yoga in front of a man. I think I will just wait." This exact scenario has taken place right before my eyes numerous times. As you can see, if this question was *deafeared*, or answered with a question, this would have never become a problem.

Ask for the Sale Five Times!

One of the most effective turnovers in sales is to "go ask them one more time." The reason is, people give up. People change their mind. Sixty percent of all sales that are made in the world are done so after the fifth closing objection. It is true. Count how many objections or concerns you field while you are with your next couple of guests. I bet it is more than just two or three. Here is something to think about while handling these numerous objections:

- If you give up on the first objection (some salespeople do) you will miss 90 percent of all sales you could have made if you could have handled the five objections.

- If you give up on the second concern (a lot of salespeople do), you will miss 80 percent of all sales you could have made if you could have handled the five objections.

- If you give up on the third concern (most salespeople do), you will miss 70 percent of all sales that could have been made if only you could have handled the five objections.

- Give up on the fourth concern (do *you*?), you are missing 60 percent of all the people you could have helped if you just would have asked one more time.

You get the point. If you do not have the ability to make your guests feel comfortable, you do not have the ability to build rapport, or you do not use the steps outlined in the "overcoming objections" section, you will never have the ability to make your guests feel comfortable enough to where you are able to field several objections without offending them. Remember, sometimes you just have to take the long way around. This may mean getting up from the table and clearing the air, or going back out on the workout floor and re-explaining some of the facilities. Change the scenery for a while. Change the entire subject and try talking for a while about something that has nothing to do with joining the yoga center. If you are too direct, you will never get to objection number five. Number five is the magic number. It separates the men from the boys, the girls from the women.

After Asking Questions, Shut Up!

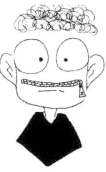

The reason we ask questions is to give the guest the opportunity to think of the answer. If you do not wait for the answer, you are giving them the answer. When you do this, you are not letting the guests think on their own, and they are certainly not being closed. You must be patient, ask a question, and give the guests as much time as they need to answer the question. When they answer the question, be ready with the next question. Do not ever interrupt your guest; the first one to talk loses the battle! Below is an example of a typical situation where you need to ask questions, wait for a response and then be ready for another question.

For Example:

"Mary, why did you come to the studio today?" "I want to lose weight." *"Mary, if you do not mind me asking, you look great to me, why did you want to lose weight?"* "I just saw a picture of myself, and I cannot believe how much weight I have gained." *"How did you feel when you saw that picture, Mary?"* "I couldn't believe it! I decided right then and there that tomorrow I was going to lose fifteen pounds." *"Mary, if I could show you the perfect program to help you lose weight and feel great about yourself in the shortest time*

possible, would you be interested in getting started today?" "Absolutely!" *"Mary, did you want to go ahead with the membership that included our one-on-one yoga and nutrition or would you just prefer to go with our basic membership today?"* "I will take the Yoga and nutrition." *"Welcome to the studio!"*

Closing Types

The Verbal Closing: *"If I could, would you"*

Of all the closes I can think of, this one is still one of the best. It is, "If I could, would you." This means that if I could get that for you today would you want to get started. You always want to be two steps ahead of the other salespeople.

For Example:

"You know, we used to have this deal. I do not know if I can still get it for you, but I can talk to my manager. I do not know if he will go for it, but if I could *talk to him and see if I could get that for you,* would you *be interested in getting started today?"*

In many cases you will show the potential member your membership options and they will say they want to think about it. What you need to do is mention the deal that was just available, but has since expired. Then you can offer the "if I could, would you" close.

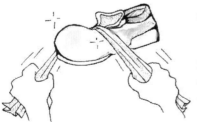

Two sales, One guest

This close I am going to tell you in story form. I see so many sales counselors make the mistake of not taking the opportunity of turning one sale into two or three sales. This happens because of a very simple reason: They never ask for it. I travel back and forth from the United States to Taiwan on a regular basis. Since I live in Nevada, I usually have a lay over in San Francisco. There is a young boy there who is great at shining shoes. He is a master at his trade. He puts a lot of flare into the art of shoe shining. As I arrive at the San Francisco Airport, I see that he is working. I go over to him and ask him how much it is for a shoeshine. He replies by saying, "All of the other shine boys charge $2.50. If you want a shine from me, it is going to cost you $3. It is a little more but I guarantee you, you will know where that extra 50 cents went." Then he turns his eyes down towards my shoes, and he says, "Those look like a pair of expensive shoes." I say, "Yes, they are. They cost a lot of money." Then he replies to me, "Why don't you buy a cheaper pair of shoes, like ones from discount shoe stores?" I respond by saying, "Quality is important to me. I believe you get what you pay for." He looks me in the eyes, smiles, and responds by saying, "Then I guess you want to have your shoes shined by me." I smile and take a seat in the chair. He opens up his box and starts to shine my shoes. Each time the towel hits my shoes, it makes a popping sound. He has perfected this trick over the thousands of shoes he must have polished.

He spins the towel and hums and appears as if he is singing a song with the friction and popping coming from the towel. He then looks down at the bottom of my shoes and says to me, "These are Italian leather shoes, and I must admit they are some of the nicest I have ever seen." As he comes to the finish, I can see he has done an excellent job shining my shoes. He looks at me and he says, "You know I have something in my box that they made just for expensive Italian shoes just like these. It may cost you 50 cents more, but your shoeshine will last twice as long. Do you want to go with the Italian lotion or did you just want me to finish up with the cheap stuff?" By now, I am sure you can guess my answer. Just by the way that he phrased his questions and the confidence he did it with, I was sold. A professional salesman being closed by a boy.

He then does something that most experienced salespeople often forget to do. He asks me how long my lay over will be. I respond by saying that I will be in the airport for another couple of hours before taking off for my home. He then asks me if I have to dress up for work every day. I respond by saying, "Yes, unfortunately, I have to wear a suit and tie to work." The boy then responds by saying, "Do you wear the same pair of shoes every day?" I say, "No, I have different color shoes for the different suits that I wear." As I see the wheels in his head turning, he looks at me and says, "If you have other shoes with you, I will be willing to shine them as well. Not only that, but I will be willing to put the expensive Italian lotion on them for free, sound fair?" Without giving me the time to respond, he follows up by saying, "Leave your shoes here for me, go grab something to eat, and they will be ready in 20 minutes." Whether I say yes to this or whether I say no is not the point. The point is that he asked. He turns one sale into three, and he adds 50 cents with the lotion. I am sure that not every person says yes, but if 25 percent of the people do, he increases his sales by a large percentage. Do not forget to *up-sell*. Who says you can't learn a lot from a child?

Are you aware of the fact that McDonald's Corp. increases their sales 25 percent by simply asking one question: "Would you like fries or a coke with that?" They took it even one step further by asking people if they would like to "SuperSize" their fries and cokes. They take the sale one step further by changing their menus from having all the different foods listed on the menu to having meal deals on the menu. Instead of having to pick just the hamburger or just the french-fries, they all come together in a meal for one low price.

The Lost Sale Close

The *lost sale* close is one you can use when your guest is in the parking lot. It is a last ditch effort when every thing else has failed. It starts with first letting the guest know that you are aware they are not going to join the studio today but you were just letting them know that this is how you earn a living. Tell them that their feedback is important to you improving your craft and ask them some questions.

For Example:

"What did I do wrong? I must have done something wrong? I can't help anyone get started. I just want to help people and no one wants to help themselves. Is it me? Is something wrong with me? Did I do something to offend you? Maybe I am just not cut out to help people. Maybe those other used car salesmen inside were right.

Maybe I should quit being so nice and just start taking people's money. Forget about their goals and dreams."

I know, I know, it is a pretty low move. It is also pretty shameless. But, believe it or not, this method does work from time to time. Hopefully you do not find yourself in any situations where you have to resort to a tactic like this. If you do find yourself in that situation, it is good to have a script ready.

The Alternate Choice

The *alternate choice* is what we do when we show prospects all of the different membership options and then say, "Would you want to go with option one or would you prefer option two? Out of the different options which one are you leaning towards? Did you want to start today or would tomorrow be better for you? Do you want your membership with an instructor or without an instructor?" The alternate choice is a simple and effective close. In sales, you will learn that if you give somebody two choices they are going to take one of them. "Did you want to go with cash, check or credit card?" It has been around forever and works in all types of businesses. Learn it and get used to it because you will see that you will probably use this close as much as any other.

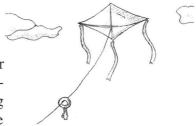

The Ben Franklin Close

This close is especially good for closing a one-on-one yoga membership. This close involves developing a plus *vs.* minus system. This close does not necessarily have to be a yoga center close. It can be used for anything that you are trying to sell. What really matters is that you have the positives and the negatives of why the potential member should make a decision. It works very well and do not be afraid if it takes a while. Do not be afraid that you may have to go through a little bit of a process in order to make this happen.

Ben Franklin was a smart man, one of the founders of our country and, obviously, he had to make a number of complicated decisions. Whenever Ben Franklin had to make a difficult decision he would list the positives and the negatives of why he should make that decision. He would make a list of all the reasons why he should do it and all the reasons why he should not do it. Based on the positives against the negatives, he would weigh it out and decide if he should make the decision or wait for a while before deciding. If the positives outweighed the negatives, he would make that decision and *vice versa*.

For example, what you need to do is write the answers to questions given by the customer on a piece of paper. Title one side of the paper, *Positives* and the other side of the paper, *Negatives*. Ask the customer, "What positives do you think will come from you becoming more healthy and losing weight?" The answers will vary and include such positives as health, looking good, lower blood pressure, feeling better, strengthen the heart, energy, stamina, and more. If they do not come up with enough give them a couple of more positives so you can fill up that column. Do not give them too many because you want them to see their answers on the paper. After writing down about 10 to 12 positives, move over to the negatives. Ask the customer, "What are some of the negatives you can see by getting in shape and improving your health?" The funny thing about the question is that there is no acceptable answer to it. Whatever you do, do not help them fill out this side of the paper. They will have a hard time finding any answers so do not give them any. You will receive answers such as, "I don't have the time" or "I don't have the money," two of the easiest objections to overcome. That is about it. You have not only showed them that the positives outweigh the negatives, you have also uncovered a couple of objections. Your next step is to read back all of the positives and then the negatives. Your closing question will be something like, "Mary, wouldn't you agree that sacrificing an average of one hour of your time and around $1 a day is a small price to pay to be able to live longer, look better, have more energy, lower you blood pressure, sleep better, and more?" (Simply read back their positives.)

You have now made it obvious that their objections have been squashed underneath the pressure of all of the positives they are going to receive. You have built value within the product and shown that they need to listen to you to get what they need. The only way to get all of the positives is to enroll in the studio. Once they have seen that, they find it hard to say no because it is simply not a logical answer. It takes a little longer but it is well worth it.

Motivational Speaker

"Mary, last week I went to a seminar, it was put on by a motivational speaker. He explained that the reason people are unhappy with their life is that they worry about the little things and they do not take care of the big things. He said and I think you will agree, that there are four major areas in your life. If you take care of these four areas, then the rest of your life will be enjoyable. The four things were your relationships (friends, family, and loved ones), financial stability, spirituality, and your health. He explained that these four things affected each other. Having no friends or family could affect your health. Having poor health could affect your job. Having no spirituality could affect your ability to care or have a meaning in life. Now, Mary, I do not know if the motivational speaker was right or wrong, but I think you would agree with me that without your health, nothing else really matters."

The Negative Take-Away Close

I found that this close works extremely well with a person that shows little interest or emotion. You have to find something in this individual that will stimulate action. I found that sometimes the only way to do this is by taking something away. You may find that your guest says that they are not really interested in joining the studio. They are not really interested in exercise, and they never thought about working out before. It is going to be hard for you to gain commitment if you cannot get your guest's attention. You may simply state that it is OK even if they wanted to join the studio today; it would be impossible for you to sign them up. Tell them that unfortunately, at this time, the studio is full of members that care about being healthy. You may recommend putting them on a waiting list and giving them a call back when there is an opening for enrollment. This may spark something in them that makes them want something they cannot have. This guest may be using this technique to try to get you to beg them to join. When you do not show interest, they will be surprised. This will cause them to loosen up on their objections and force him or her to show an interest to get what you will not give him or her. Often times, the prospect will try to buy their way through the waiting list.

Magic Potion

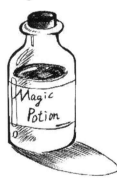

I use this close quite often for the person that believes that there are shortcuts to becoming healthy. Trendy diets, weight loss retreats, starving, steroids, all of these are worthless with out exercise and a good diet, yet people still waste their time trying them. You have to use a little bit of imagination, and you have to have somewhat of a good rapport with your guest. Ask your guest to think of a time when they were in the best shape of their life. Make them think about the time when they felt great, looked great, and people would comment on their accomplishments. Then I would pick up a cup or a bottle of white out and I would look at the guest and say, "What if I had a magic potion, and that magic potion you could drink and in the morning when you wake, you would have the perfect body? If I had a potion like that, how much do you think I would be able to sell it for?" You can ask your guest, "If I had a potion like that, how much will you be willing to pay for it?" Your guest may respond by saying, "That would be priceless. You can sell it for any amount." I respond by saying, "So you would agree that your body is also priceless? You and I both know there is no quick fix, there is no magic potion. Believe me, if there was, Oprah Winfrey would not be overweight.

The only way for you to have the perfect body is to adjust your life-style to include your priceless body."

The Magic Potion close works to get the guest to understand that there is no easy way to losing weight and maintaining their health. This close must be done with whom you have built a strong rapport. If you try it with someone who you do not have a good rapport with, they will not follow along and will miss the point of the presentation.

The Only Car You Will Ever Have

When I first started in sales, this close was one used by a good friend of mine. Personally, I have never used it. But it seemed to work very well for him. He would simply ask the guest a series of questions to make the guest realize how important health and yoga was. He would compare the person's body to an automobile. He would state, "Mary, I want you to imagine, you are living in a foreign country. And in this country, there is a rule; the rule is that you are only going to have one car in your entire lifetime. The rule is put in place to teach people to take care of things and be responsible. On your 21st birthday, you are given your one automobile to have for your lifetime. Would you change the oil in your automobile? Would you keep your automobile clean? Would you put the best gasoline in it? Would you put the protection on the rubber and leather? I am sure you would agree with me, if you were only going to have one automobile for the rest of your life, it would be of the highest priority to take care of it. Wouldn't you agree? Mary, the reason I ask you these questions is in relation to your body. You only get one body; you will never ever have a chance to get another one. I think you would agree that having one body is more important than having one car."

This is a very successful close. The entire time you are working to gain the agreement of your guest. Once they have realized the point or the correlation between the story and their body, it becomes almost irrational for them to say no. Again, this must be done with a person you have built a strong rapport with. If you do not, much like the Magic Potion close, they will not gain the significance of it.

Benefits Not Bashing

One of the most important techniques used in sales today is selling on just benefits. How is our product going to benefit the customer? Why it is important for the customer to need the product? How does our product differ from other products? All of these questions need to be addressed before you are going to make a successful sale. The goal is to cut down on everything but the pure benefits. It is important to use our three-step method (outlined in the Tours chapter), statement of fact, two to three questions and a tie-down.

For Example:

"Mary, now I have explained the benefits of our one-on-one yoga program, I think you would agree that no other yoga center can offer a program to compare with ours." It is important not to knock other yoga centers; it can ruin your credibility. When a guest talks about the benefits of another studio, I simply agree and say *"Mary, No. #1 Yoga is a very nice studio, and I think you would agree that it has a very good price. But what I would like to do is take a moment of your time to tell you the benefits of our facility, as well as the best price, and let you make the decision for yourself, sound fair?"*

By doing this, you are keeping the member interested in your studio. You are allowing them to make their own decision but asking them in a way that only the answer "yes" will benefit them. Remember, you are there to make them happy. If you are looking out for their interests and trying to find benefits for them, they will appreciate it and you will have a strong rapport.

The "Thinking About It" Close

This objection is at the tip of every customer's tongue if they are going to give one. If a guest gives you this objection, they are in a situation where they are searching for a way out of committing, most likely to try to avoid spending money. It is what we call a "secondary objection" because it is often used to hide another. When the situation arises, stay calm and remember this close.

For Example:

"I can understand you want to think about it. Other people have felt the same way that you feel. What we have found is that most people have already thought of everything there is to think about. Then what ends up happening is you go home, you walk towards the door, you pick up your mail, and you start thinking about the bills you have to pay. You go in and listen to your answering machine, turn on the TV, get busy with the dinner and kids. One thing leads to another, and all of a sudden, it is six months down the road, and you really have not gotten back around to doing what you originally had the best intentions of doing today. Every morning we wake up and have the best intentions of doing all of the things that are going to make our life better. It just seems by noon, or half way through the day, our mind has tricked our bodies into making the wrong decision, into procrastinating, waiting, or putting it off until tomorrow. I think you would agree, that the time is right, and now is the time. What better place to think about it? You have all the information that you need on the table, you have an environment that is free from distraction, and you have me here to answer all of your questions."

It is quite a bit to remember but it is the only close you are going to need in this situation. You will find that people will make objections, such as this one, just because they are afraid to commit to anything. When they are in a situation where they cannot find anything they truly object to, they will fall back on their old-reliable "I want to think about it."

"What about this? What about that? What if I could?" Close

I have found that the most effective close is just offering the guest different options until you find one that works for them. Most of the time, your guest is not going to tell you the real reason they are not joining. They will come up with objections instead of telling you the real reason they are not joining the studio is you, as the professional, have not found a membership option to fit their needs. I read a great book about sales not too far back that really opened my eyes. Two salesmen wrote this book, and it only contained facts and figures on what motivated people to make a purchase.

They put hidden cameras in sales offices all over the world and studied what the key points involved in the person's final decisions were. More interestingly to me was when they focused on what the different salespeople did in different situations when confronted with different objections. The two biggest factors were No. 1, the want to be sales professional never asked for the sale, and No. 2, they could not find an option that met the customer's needs. Many salespeople today cannot close a sale because they do not understand the fact that the one or two options that they are offering are not working for the customer.

For Example:

"Mary, this membership option includes a one time upfront investment, leaving your monthly investment at only $25." "I need to think about it." *"Mary, let me ask you a question, is pre-paying your membership an option for you?"* "I still want to try it first." *"Mary, what if I could get you a short-term membership that would give you an opportunity to try the studio, as well as a little more time to see the benefits exercise will have on you?"* "That sounds a little better." *"I have a 90 day option for $120 and I have 120 day option for $200. Both of them would give you the time to see changes in your body, at the end of that time, your membership will expire. If you decide you like the studio, and you are seeing results, within the first 30 days, you can apply the total amount towards a regular membership. I think this will answer all of your concerns. Out of option 1 and option 2, which one would you be leaning towards?"* "Option 2." *"Mary, welcome to the studio. Your address? Phone number? Would you be handling your membership by cash, check or credit card?"* "Credit card." *"And you brought that with you today?"*

The example I have given above shows that Mary really did want to join. I simply had to find a membership option that elevated her concerns and met her needs. This is very common in our business. Many times it is not that the guest does not want to enroll, it is that the guest has not seen anything that they really feel comfortable with. The reason most successful studios have multiple membership options is so they can tailor to the many different needs of many different people. It is your job to find the best one for each situation.

The "Just Do It" Close

I hate to say it, but sometimes just saying the words, *"Oh, come on, just do it!"* will be motivation enough for some people to enroll. I do not know why this works, but it does. I do not know how many times this close has been used in high schools to get a under-aged kid to drink his first beer, but it just has something to do with peer pressure. The words, *"Oh, come on, just do it!"* work.

You must have a good rapport with your guest to use this one. It is playful, yet effective. Many people simply need to have somebody there to give them that extra shove to get them going.

My Grandma Close

This close works very well with senior citizens and long-time procrastinators. A lot of times you will be unable to get older people to even answer any of the questions. When this happens, I change gears and go from sales mode to story mode. I simply sit down at the table and say,

"Mary, I know that you are not interested in making a decision today. You know there is a little story I would like to tell you, it would only take a minute of your time if you do not mind. I wanted to tell you the reason I got into this business. When I was in my early 20s, I was still very active in sports and was very serious about making it to the gym on the daily basis. At the time, I was concerned with looking great and feeling great, and I truly could not understand why anyone did not exercise. At that time, I had a grandmother who was in her early 60, and was in pretty poor physical condition. She worked long hours; her diet included a steady supply of cheese, chips, coffee, cigarettes and aspirin. Several times a week, I would stop by her house on my way to the gym and raid her refrigerator. On my way out, I would ask her, 'Grandma, why don't you go to the gym with me today? There are lots of other people there just like you, and they

feel great about their exercise programs.' She would always respond by saying, 'I am busy', or 'Not today, I will go with you tomorrow.' She would give me every excuse in the book. As the years went by, she seemed to have less energy, more health problems, and an over-all, lackluster outlook on life. So finally one day, I walked in her house, I put her in a headlock, I literally dragged her, kicking and scratching into a yoga class with me. After taking a 15-minute swim and some light resistance training, my grandmother had seemed to be reborn. She spoke to some of the other seniors in the club, and they gave her a schedule for the senior yoga classes. After leaving the facility, she felt energy and vigor that she had not felt in years. My grandmother has continued on an exercise program three days a week for the past seven years. If you were to ask her about her physical condition, she would tell you she feels better at 70 than she felt at 40. Mary, if I let you leave the studio today without a membership, I would be going against everything that my grandmother believes was the best decision she ever made. She still reminds me of the day that I dragged her to the car and dragged her into the gym, and it reminds me of the joy of helping someone, like yourself, do what you know you should do right now!"

Overcoming Objections

I am going to give you two or more ways to overcome each of the objections.

"Spouse (I want to talk husband or wife, Mom or dad.")

Option 1

"I want to talk to my wife" "you want to talk to your wife?" "Yes we have an agreement whenever we do anything in regard to money we talk it over!" "I can understand that I am married too and this is a big decision. I know you wouldn't even be considering talking to your wife if you weren't **very** serious. Let me ask you one question other than talking to your wife is there any thing else holding you back from getting started to day?" "No." "Let me ask you this Larry, if the yoga membership was twenty dollars for the entire year would you be able to make a decision today with out your wife." "Yes." "So you can spend money without talking to your wife, just not a lot of money, is it the upfront enrollment or the monthly investment that is too much." "It is the total price!" "So if I could talk to my boss and get your total price reserved with a small deposit and you could go home and talk to your wife would that work for you?" "Yes." "How much could you put down today to hold this price?" "Half." "Okay Larry let me go talk to my boss." "Larry how do you normally handle your business, cash check or credit card?" "Credit card." "You brought that with you today?"

Option 2

You go call your husband and see if he will let you get started on a yoga program, and I will call my wife and see if it is okay for me to sell the membership to you."

Option 3

"Your wife is going to say no?" "No, my wife isn't going to say no." "Well, she doesn't care, she probably won't want you to spend money." "Is she is going say yes?" "If you are so sure your wife will say yes, then you really don't still need to ask her?"

Option 4

"Your body has nothing to do with any other person other than you. Your husband/wife cannot workout for you or tell you not to work out. Your body is yours, and it is 100 percent your decision. Buying a car or a house is different, because it is communal property. Your body belongs to you and it is your decision if you want to be healthier or feel good about the way you look. No other person can make that decision, wouldn't you agree?"

"Shop around. (I want to go see other yoga studios)"

Option 1

List of other studios: "Let me give you a list of studios to shop that will make your job easier. These studios are a lot cheaper they do not have air-conditioning, but I think they will work for you."

Option 2

Refund option: "I can give you three days to shop around. If for any reason you find any studios you like better, come back to get a full refund, and I can still give you a discount by starting today. There is nothing to lose!"

Option 3

If it is over the telephone: *"I want you to go to all the other studios in town, make sure you take notes about the different price options and services that are provided by the other studios. Then, I want you to come to our studio with the information. I will prove to you that our studio can beat any other studio when it comes to the services that we provide. Not only that, but I will also beat any studios price. I think you would agree this is the right way to make the most educated decision. Would morning or evening be best for you?"*

"Time. (I don't have it)"

Option 1

I usually quickly respond by saying, "you don't have time not to!"

Option 2

John, you have already made an incredible investment in regards to the time and amount of money that you have put aside for exercise, if time is a concern, I can show you that I specialize in programs that give you more results in less time. Now you will have more time.

"I want to try it out. (I will join after I use my pass)"

Option 1

John, I understand that you want to try it on your own, I also understand that you have had success in the past. Exercise is a relatively new concept and fitness in regards to what works and what does not. Some of the new information that I have to offer can help you get results quicker and easier and I'm sure if you are like everyone else, you would like to make your workouts quicker, easier, and more effective.

Option 2

This objection is hard to overcome, because it is a real objection. The first thing you should do is to make sure that a pass is not sitting on the table. Never leave your passes anywhere but at the front desk. There are a few variations of the second option available for you.

"Mary, you are looking for permanent results with a temporary 10 visit pass. I think you would agree with me that your membership does not meet your goals. It would be unfair for me as yoga professional to set you up for failure."

Option 3

"Mary, it sounds like you have some very serious goals. I want you to stop for a second, and think about this. You wake up in the morning, and you look at yourself in the mirror, you are extremely proud of the results that you and your instructor have achieved. In three months, you have lost 20 pounds. And all of your clothes are a little bit looser than they used to be. People have been commenting you on how good you look, and then your self-image improves. Once you achieve results, Mary, how soon would you like to go back to your original shape?" "I would not want to go back to my original shape." *"So I think I will be correct in saying that you are looking for long-term results."* "Yes."

Option 4

John, when I was in my early 20's, I decided to take up golf. I went out and bought an expensive set of golf clubs, and despite the pro shop advice, I refused having a pro give me some pointers. In time, I developed a very interesting new system for making the ball curve when I hit it. When I finally decided to go in and see a professional to make an adjustment, it was extremely difficult for me to change my bad habits. If I had of learned to play golf the right way in the beginning, I would have been well adjusted by this time. I implore you not to make the same mistake or pick-up the same bad habits that I did.

"I want to think about it. (I will be back)"

Option 1

"I can give you three days to shop around. If for any reason you find any other product that offers better reliability or you like better, come back to get a full refund, and I can still give you a discount by starting today. There is nothing to lose!"

Option 2

"Mr. Prospect, you want to think about it? I can understand you want to think about it. I understand how you feel. Other people have felt the same way, but what we have found is that by joining on a membership today, it will be the best decision you will ever make in your life. Other than thinking about it, is there anything else to stop you from getting started today?" "No." "May I ask you a question? How many days are you going to need to think about?" "Two days." "What if I could give you two days to think about it, and still give you a discount on your yoga classes by starting up today? I could give you a discount today and you would have three days to decide to keep your membership or get a refund. Sound fair?"

Option 3

"Mary, how long have you been thinking about joining a studio?" "One year."

"Do you still need to think about it? If thinking about it could get you in shape, you would be Mr. America by now. If thinking about money each day could help me save money, I would be rich by now.

*Thinking about it won't make anything happen. The worse decision
you can make, is to make a decision, to not make a decision."*

"Group/friends" "I have a friend and we want to take yoga together."

Option 1

It is true taking yoga with a friend can offer some great benefits, in most cases I found that in modern day society, with jobs and families, and all the things going on, sometimes being consistent with a partner can be impossible. Why don't we get you started on our special rate, and if your friend is interested, they can join on a v.i.p. guest pass.

Option 2

"You know I can understand, Mary, you want to wait for your friend before you start your membership. There are a million reasons that we can come up with to not get started on a membership today. And believe me, I hear them all. I am very concerned with you getting started today, and I do not want your friends' excuses to become yours. What if I can give you a discounted rate on our membership options? Not only that, but I will be willing to ask my manager to put your friend on our VIP guest list. What that means to you, Mary, is that when you join the studio today, not only will you get a great price, but your friend can come in within the next two days and receive a two-week free trial membership as well as a guaranteed rate of exactly what you paid. Mary, if I can ask my manager to put your friend on our VIP guest list, would you want to get started today?"

Option 3

"No, if you come back later with your friends I will not be able to guarantee the same deal. But what I can try to do is give you a good discount today, right now, and if your friends come in and join within 30 days, I will try and get them the same deal."

Option 4

Not only do I specialize in 1-on-1 personal training and nutrition, but I also specialize in group training sessions. If you would be interested, I might be able to talk to my boss and include a program that would teach you and your friend how to train together and how to accomplish your goals in the shortest amount of time possible. If I can talk to my boss and teach you and your friend how to benefit from group training, how would you handle your business: cash, credit card, or check?

"It's too expensive."

Option 1

You can break it down to the ridiculous, most of the time it will be. "*Your membership is $20 per month, how much too much is it?*" "It is $5 too much." "*So $5 is stopping you from joining the studio today?*" "Yes." "*Five dollars divided by 30 days equals 16 cents per day, so 16 cents per day is stopping you from becoming healthier? Don't you think your health and happiness is worth 16 cents per day?*"

Option 2

"It's too expensive" is the best objection we can get. Out of all of the other objections, it is truly the one we have the most control over. We cannot control what their husbands are going to say, cannot control how convenient the club is for them. But we certainly have control over different membership options and prices available to them. You must learn how to handle this objection with many different tactics. If you do not, you will lose a large number of potential sales. You are going to hear it, so you better start practicing for it.

Option 3

"Out of the different membership options, which one are you leaning toward?" "it's too expensive." "was it the shape up yoga package, the total fitness or the vip program that was a little more than you were looking to spend?" "*I really just think that it is a little out of my price range."* "Which one of the yoga memberships is a little bit too much, the shape up, the total fitness or the vip?" *"I really like the shape up the best but I am not ready to get started until I talk to my husband."* "Did you want to talk to your husband about the upfront investment or did you want to talk to your husband about the monthly price?" *"I want to talk to my husband about the total membership price."* "What if I could talk to my boss and get you payment options so that the total membership price is more convenient for you, would that make you feel more comfortable?" *"Yes."* If I could talk to my boss and break your membership up into payments, would you want to handle your business by cash or credit card?" *"Credit card."* "You brought that with you today."

Exclusivity price objection

"Mary, I can understand that you think the studio is a little bit more than you would like to pay. Let's think about this for a minute. Mary, did you buy the cheapest car you could find? Did you buy the cheapest watch you could find? Did you buy the cheapest house you could find? The answers to these questions are probably no, and I think if I was to answer for you, you would say that buying the cheapest thing does not always mean that you are getting the two most important things, quality and value. It is true that we do charge a little bit more for our studio. The reason why is that we care about exclusivity. Mary, would you want to be a member of a studio where any person with $20 in their pockets can come in off the street and join? You seem like a person that understands value, and I think you also understand by paying a little bit more, you will also be getting a little bit more. You can see the value in that, right Mary?"

"It's not convenient"

It is a true objection, so sometimes it is very difficult to overcome.

"We have a membership for people who live far away. However, it only allows you to use the studio four to six times a month." "I would

want to use it more than that." "*So the studio is convenient enough for you to make it down more than six times a month?*" "Yes." "*Where you live is not going to change, but if it was not convenient for you, you would not be here. If there were a more convenient studio for you, you would already be their member. Is the studio convenient enough for you.*" "Yes." "*Welcome to the studio.*"

Chapter 22

ONE-ON-ONE YOGA

The one-on-one yoga department may be one of the fastest grow-ing areas of yoga centers today. The most successful members of the studio are the ones who have personal instructors. People from all walks of life can benefit from one-on-one yoga. A large percentage of top athletes and major actors work with professional instructors to achieve maximum results. Always remember, getting results is the key to our business. It is important that you under-stand a successful system for learning how to sell one-on-one yoga. I believe the first step in selling one-on-one yoga is that you must understand what it is that the instructors do. The second step is that you have to develop a presentation that builds value into this results oriented program. The fourth step is presenting different price op-tions and the fifth step is closing the sale.

Step One: Understanding What It Is the Instructors Do

The instructors do *goal setting* for the members, achievable goals and body measurements, so everything is down on paper. That way the member can follow their improvement. They also focus on other important areas such as *food intake*, working with the food that members like to eat. If the plan includes the foods that the member likes to eat, it makes the program more convenient for them and easier to follow. The instructors also cover the benefits of *supple-mentation*, alternate foods and vitamins that may help get results; *accountability*, making sure that the members show up to exercise; *consistency,* making sure the members workout on a consistent basis about three and four times a week; *motivation,* getting the most out of every single workout. Motivation is needed to hit your goal. The plan also includes the use of *proper techniques*, to avoid injuries and manipulating every set and rep to get the optimal benefit. And *program design* designs everything for the individual so they achieve long-term results and a lifetime education of yoga.

Step Two: The Benefits of One-on-one yoga

The benefits of one-on-one yoga are endless, but I will single out a few: better, longer life through exercise; education you can take with you for a lifetime; better self-esteem; impact on your personal relationships; better performance at work; more energy; healthy meal plans; and lower stress levels. This is just a portion of the benefits. The possibilities are endless.

Step Three: Building the Benefits through the Presentation

I personally recommend that you copy the script from one of the top personal instructors in your company. It will most likely resemble a script like the one I recommended previously in the greeting and introduction chapter. I worked with an outstanding instructor who lent his script to all the salespeople to help them increase one-on-one yoga sales. It was three pages long and it took me a month to memorize, but it worked great. The first month I used the presentation my sales went through the roof. I sold $9,000 in one-on-one yoga in just the first month I learned this presentation. It focuses on building the benefits on the training program and helps guests to understand what they are paying $60 dollars an hour for. Remember, you cannot show somebody in one hour what it is exactly the personal instructor is going help them accomplish. Therefore, you have to paint a picture in the person's mind of exactly what benefits they are going to receive from the service. If the benefits outweigh the money, your member will be willing to make the trade, money for results.

Step Four: Price Presentation

You should have a price presentation that has several different options of price and programs. There should be a program to fit every budget from executives to students. The programs should be able to meet the needs of all individual goals. There are many different goals that the members will have. A few of the most common are weight loss programs, weight gain programs, re-hab programs for injuries, toning and firming programs, and a basic introduction to a yoga program. Your studio should have packages priced from $50 to $5,000 and 3 sessions to 50 sessions. These are the standard for pricing and sessions that most studios have. There should also be a price presentation. The presentations may vary so you should check with the instructors at your particular studio.

Step Five: Closing the Sale

Your perspective member will give you the exact same objections you will get when you are trying to sell a membership. You will hear everything from "I want to think about it" to "I need to talk it over with my husband." Your closing techniques should be the same as with a membership and you should do everything you can from "TOing" to "price drops" to "post dated checks." You will always find a time to ask the question: "If I can get you a good deal, would you want to purchase one-on-one yoga today?" You have to realize that one-on-one yoga accounts for 30 percent of sales in yoga centers today. People are in the gym and are willing to spend their money and their time because they want to see results. It is the results that you have to sell. One-on-one yoga is the most efficient method the members can use to achieve those results. This is a very important aspect of what we do and if you cannot master this area, you will never be a complete professional, and you will be left behind in our industry.

Chapter 22a

ONE-ON-ONE YOGA PRESENTATION

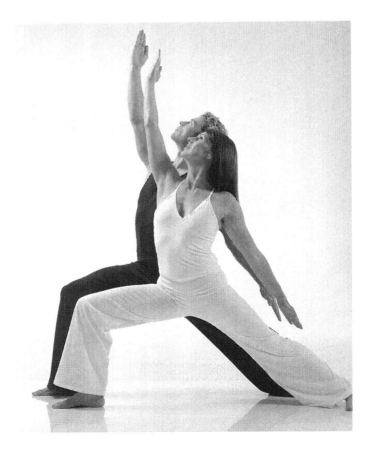

Memorize, Utilize, Maximize Your Success

Mr. Prospect, the starting point of one-on-one yoga is goal setting. It's about setting a target of what you want to achieve because if you can't see your target, how are you going to hit it? Right?

Have you ever set goals before? What your instructor is going to do is set challenging, believable, achievable goals within a specific time frame, then put them down on paper so now they become measurable.

Proper food intake also plays a big role. About 60 to 70 percent of your success in the studio is going to be from the things you eat outside the studio. How is your diet right now? How many times per day are you eating? What your instructor is going to do is have you bring in two to three days of your current food intake. Do you think that might be something your able to do?

The third aspect of ensuring your results is the accountability factor. What that means to you is that you will be much more likely to come down to the facility and have a quality workout when you have an appointment set with a certified professional. If for any reason you don't make it in your instructor will be calling you saying we can't accomplish your goals if your not here! Can you see how that will benefit you?

And accountability over time works out to be consistency. We know that in anything, if we are not consistent, we are not going to be successful. So your instructor ensures that you adhere to your regular exercise program in order to accomplish your goals. We recommend that you meet with your instructor two to three days per week for optimal results. How many days will you be able to commit to working with your instructor?

Now, motivation ties into this because your instructor instills in you a greater degree of commitment to accomplishing your goals. Motivation is the difference between accelerated results and just kind of moving along at a slow rate, and I'm sure you're like everyone else and you prefer results sooner rather than later, right?

Proper technique also plays a big role. First of all to avoid injury, and secondly, if you aren't doing things correctly you're not going to get the optimum benefits for the equipment and your time.

Now, the "one-on-one" in one-on-one yoga comes in with program design. This involves your instructor designing a customized program for you and how your body responds so you maximize every rep, set, and minute in the facility to achieve your goals.

Price Prezo

Now, Mr. Prospect, normally a session of is going to run you $70 per session. But what the company has done to make it more affordable for you as a member is they have grouped them into packages to suit your specific needs. As you can see, the more you show that you are committed to achieving your yoga goals, the rate per session goes down. The first option is great; it's what I call the starter package. It gives you some time and knowledge and how to apply it in the studio so you can take it and be successful.

Now, Mr. Prospect, I'm going to skip to this package for now and move on to what I call our accelerated results package. As you can see, when you enroll in a 32-session package with the instructor the rate drops all the way down to $49 per session. The great thing is that this is the one that our most successful members are a part of. This package will give you the benefits of being dialed in to achieving your yoga goals through a longer-term commitment and you take advantage of the lowest rate. So you can see that this package is obviously the best value. Right? You will really see substantial changes in your body with this package.

Now, I skipped the 16-session package for a very simple reason, Mr. Prospect. This is the most popular package when people enroll in the program on a first-time basis. It's the one that most people in your position go with. It's great because you get an obviously reduced rate and a substantial period of time to work with the instructor and experience the true benefits of the program. You will begin to recognize the effect of your progress in terms of results in this time.

Now, I will back you in any decision that you make today towards accomplishing your goals. Out of the different options, which one would you be leaning towards?

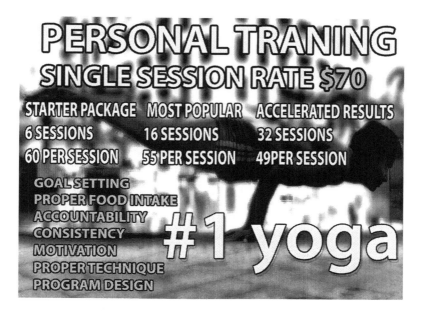

Chapter 23

HOW AND WHEN

TO *T.O.*

TO stands for *take over*. It is one of the most effective ways to sell a membership. The reason is that when you sell a membership, a lot of things that are going on at the table are non-verbal. I can look at someone's face and recognize when they are scared, not comfortable, in a hurry, not interested, or just want to come in and join. You should be able to tell if that person is in a hurry or should be able to adjust to these different reactions. This is what TOing is going to teach you. TOing is going to teach you what to say and when to say it and how to react to each guest differently. Usually when I am training new salespeople, I will make them get up at least five times from the table during each sales presentation.

For example:

"I will be right back, let me grab the price sheet/business card so I can find the answer for you. Will you please hold on for a moment? Let me go grab a pen / calculator."

The person is not going to leave. The reason I ask new salespeople to do this is because I want to be involved as a manager in the sales process. I want them to inform me as to what is happening at the table. Some salespeople go through the whole sales presentation having a pass sitting on the table. Getting up gives you the time and space to get advice or see how other people are selling their memberships. In some ways it is a lot like sports where teams use a timeout to stop something that is not going well or to gain momentum. You can only learn so much from listening to yourself talk. I love to sit in on sales presentations, so I can learn new things. I want to be able to learn how the other people do it. I want to know what they do differently. I want to add their strengths to my arsenal.

What is lost when you don't TO? You have lost a chance to learn. You have lost a chance to make more money. You have lost a chance to close a sale. All these things are lost when you do not TO. When I was a new yoga counselor, I asked people to TO for me all of the time. The number one rule of the TO. is you *cannot talk!* You cannot say anything. Listen, watch, learn, and feel the energy. The only time you should talk is when the guest tells a lie to the person who is TOing for you. Again, make sure that your guest is sitting down. You will never sell a membership if your guest is standing up. If you have not practiced how to get a guest to sit down, you are not going to make many sales. Here are some basic rules when TOing.

Rule 1: It is better to TO too early than too late. Do not wait until the guest is leaving, standing up, or totally upset before you TO.

Rule 2: If you are a new yoga counselor, I recommend that you TO before you give the price. That way your manager will be able to gain the commitment from the guest before showing the price.

Rule 3: TO to your manager, or the top closer in your studio. These are the people you stand to learn the most from.

Rule 4: Do not be afraid to get up. If your guest gives you an objection that you cannot overcome, get up and regroup. (*"Hold on just a second, I will be right back."*)

Rule 5: Make sure the person TOing for you stays until the completion of the sale. The person may feel like the deal was with the person TOing for you, and may bring up new objections once they leave. (Many sales are lost because of this mistake.)

Rule 6: Make sure that your company is on the same page when it comes to giving information. The last thing you would want to happen is for the person doing a TO to give different information than you just gave.

Rule 7: The most important rule: *You never open your mouth until you know what the shot is*! This refers to making sure the person that is doing the TO is aware of what is going on and does not come in and destroy your sale. A briefing prior to the take over will ensure this does not happen

Rule 8: Last but not least never ever talk. Once the TO has begun you have given up your right to talk.

Chapter 24

POST SALE

The post sale involves everything after you sell the membership. Many future opportunities are lost if you do not plant the simple seeds that can bring a flow of traffic from all of the memberships you have sold. If history has taught us anything, it is that you have to replace everything you take. If all of the lumberjacks in the world simply planted one seed next to each tree they cut down, we would have ample forests for them to work in today.

The same is true when you sell a membership. You can either tell the person that just signed up that you can give them one free month for every member they bring in to you, or simply plant the seed by saying, *"This is how I make a living, so if you want to purchase anything at the studio, please go through me. And I will make sure that you get the best price."* The post sale will also include making one-on-one yoga appointments, and if your membership agreement is like mine, it includes an area for buddy referrals, which I will go into more later on. Remember, if you can plant three seeds for every member you sign up, your member base will do all of your prospecting for you. I had a policy at my studio where every member that signed up, if within 60 days, could bring in five new enrollees, I would give that person one year for free. Although we had this policy, most salespeople would not mention it. I think you would agree that one year is well worth it for five new members. Make sure to have your general manager or sales manager check all of your deals before the new member leaves.

Chapter 25

TELEPHONE SKILLS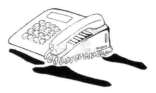

Most new salespeople hate or fear the phone. The reason for this is that most people have no experience in sales and, therefore, fear or hate sales. I talked to you earlier about the fact that a doctor trains eight or nine years before going in to surgery and a lawyer spends seven or eight years before going into a court room; but sales is an equally difficult job. Most people are put on the telephone or in a situation where they are told to get people into the studio and not given one bit of training. There are several books written on how to properly use telephones. There are also various movies that focus on the art of telephone sales or telemarketing. I suggest you read some of these books or watch a few of these films.

There are many people out there that have the skill to take people for everything they own just by using a telephone. This skill is so amazing that an unethical person can set up telephone rooms and make thousands of dollars in only a couple of days. The telephone can be so dangerous when used improperly or for the wrong reasons. There are many laws and restrictions in the United States that prevent boiler room tactics. I watched a sting operation in Chicago, where the authorities were trying to catch crooked telemarketers and telephone rip-off artists. An ad was placed in the newspaper by these authorities and then several suspected individuals were hired. They began by having the hired individuals call older men and women telling them that they had won a large sum of money. First they needed to pay the taxes to the IRS before receiving their prizes. Within the first day, literally within minutes, they had taken in thousands of dollars without using anything more than a telephone.

Selling Yoga

The telephone inquiry Call should last 3 minutes Tops; if it takes longer You may be giving out Too much information!

Now that you understand how powerful the telephone can be, you must also understand that 30 to 40 percent of all business done in the world is done on a telephone, and you must be able to add this powerful tool to your arsenal. I could write a whole book just on telephone sales. Remember, you can be anyone you want on the telephone. Make it fun! Be creative! Do not sound like a yoga counselor. People do not want to talk to telemarketers, if you say "Is Mrs. Smith there?" and she replies, "This is Mrs. Smith." and you respond by saying "Mrs. Smith, how are you doing today?" You are going to sound like every other untrained telemarketer. The reason people hate telemarketers is because most of them are young, untrained, and sound absolutely ridiculous. Is anyone other than a telemarketer or bill collector going to call you by your last name?

There is an old saying: "Smile when you are on the telephone, people can hear it." It is totally true. If you make your telephone calls with no energy and no smile, this energy will be transferred to the other end of the phone. You should try to mirror and match the energy from the caller just like you do when you are selling a membership. You should sound professional and upbeat. Speak clearly and do not use slang.

People love to talk on the telephone. Some people just love to talk. Part of the reason people don't want to talk to you is because you are trying to sell them something. Most of your sales are not going to be made over the telephone. The goal of the telephone call should be to arrange to meet the person face to face. Your phone call should not be made to sound like the sale is your only goal.

Remember, if you give out too much information over the phone, the person will not be interested in coming down to see the studio. They will already have all the information they need. Control the conversation by asking questions. The person asking the questions is the person controlling the conversation. When the person on the other end of the telephone line asks how much the membership costs, you simply respond, "Are you looking for yourself, your family or

125

your friends?" You are now in control of the conversation and will continue to be in control of the conversation as long as you keep asking questions. Let the person finish their answer before moving on to the next question.

Many of your questions should stimulate the person into thinking about the benefits for themselves and the reason they came in or are interested in the studio. (What are your main yoga goals? How long have you been thinking about accomplishing these goals? When was the last time you were in good shape? How did that make you feel?) These questions will help the person to make up their own mind based on the questions that you used to stimulate their thoughts.

Remember, it is important to take notes. If you use notes from past telephone calls, it will increase your professionalism, your ability to show caring, and your ability to make the person feel like you care. An example would be on your greeting and introduction.

It is important to use an alternate choice when trying to make an appointment. Open-ended questions will leave you with "I don't know" answers. For example, "Would you be using the studio in the morning or the evening?" "Is today or tonight better for you?" "I have an opening at 6:25 or 7:15 p.m., which would you prefer?" Also remember to keep it simple (K.I.S.S.). Again, don't give out too much information. Try to avoid giving out a price, and if you do, make the price vague.

Don't forget the power of the hold button. Know how to use the hold button if you get stuck, that way you can regroup by saying, "I am sorry, could you hold for just a moment?" Then when you get back on just say "I am sorry. It's a little busy right now. The best thing for you to do is to come in to see the studio for yourself. At that time I can answer all your questions and write down all of the different membership options, sound fair?"

Chapter 26

THE TELEPHONE INQUIRY

A large percentage of our guest traffic will come from telephone inquiries. I have found that many people, when looking for a yoga center or any other type of business, will first do so by making telephone calls. The intention of the caller is to find out as much information as they can before going out and driving around. They want to narrow their choices down over the telephone and go to the studio that they think best suits their needs. It is important for your front desk, being the first contact, to leave a good impression on the caller and to record the proper information. The telephone salutation by your service desk should go as follows:

"It is a great day to get in shape at #1 yoga, how may I help you?" The caller will ask, *"How much is a membership?"* The service person will respond by telling the person, she will transfer them to the yoga membership department, but first, *"How did you hear about the studio? May I tell the membership department your name? Lastly, can I just get your telephone number in case we get disconnected? I am going to put you on hold, and our yoga department will answer all of your questions, sound fair?"*

At that point the yoga counselor will use the telephone inquiry script. At our studio, the script is taped on the telephone, and it is important that you use the script word for word and takes notes. It is important to use the telephone skills that I outlined in the telephone skills section of the book. It is important not to give out too much information. If the caller knows all the information such as price, there will be no reason for them to visit your yoga center.

It is also important not to leave gaps if you are speaking, as the caller answers your questions, you should be ready with another question. Do not sound like you are reading, and mirror and match your caller's energy. Do not get angry or frustrated. Persistence is the key. End all your attempts to book an appointment with an alternative choice (will morning or evening best for you?). This TI script has been used successfully in thousands of yoga centers; it will bring a 70 to 80 percent closing ratio. Use it, practice, and perfect it.

Chapter 26a

YOGA TI SCRIPT

1. INTRODUCTION – "THANK YOU FOR HOLDING, THIS IS _____AND WHO AM I SPEAKING WITH?"

2. HOW DID YOU HEAR ABOUT OUR STUDIO (NAME OF STUDIO)?

3. *ARE YOU INQUIRING ABOUT A MEMBERSHIP JUST FOR YOURSELF?

*HAVE YOU BEEN A MEMBER OF A STUDIO BEFORE? IF YES, WHAT DID YOU LIKE AND DISLIKE?

*WHAT ARE YOU LOOKING TO ACCOMPLISH MOST FROM A YOGA PROGRAM?

4. BUILD PRESTIGE ON THE COMPANY.

*NUMBER OF LOCATIONS.

*OUTLINE FACILITIES (TANNING, WEIGHTS, AND MORE)

*NUMBER OF YEARS IN BUSINESS THE STABILITY OF THE COMPANY.

5. BECAUSE OF THE INCREDIBLE RESPONSE FROM A RECENT AD WE ARE SHOWING THE STUDIO BY APPOINT-MENT ONLY. WHAT I WOULD LIKE TO DO IS INVITE YOU DOWN TO SEE THE STUDIO FOR YOURSELF. AT THAT TIME

I CAN WRITE DOWN ALL YOUR DIFFERENT MEMBERSHIP OPTIONS. SOUND FAIR? WHAT WOULD BE A GOOD TIME FOR YOU? TODAY OR TONIGHT?

6. MORNING OR EVENING? (GIVE TWO OPTIONS FOR TIME.)

7. MAKE THEM WRITE IT DOWN.

8. DID YOU CALL OUR 800 NUMBER OR OUR 884 NUMBER? GREAT, YOU HAVE MY NUMBER AND WHAT WAS YOUR NUMBER?

9. THANK YOU FOR CALLING. SEE YOU AT (APPT TIME.)

What to do if they won't make an appointment

1. CLOSE FOR A TENATIVE APPOINTMENT (YOU MAY HAVE SOME FREE TIME TO POP DOWN AND SEE ME.)

2. OFFER A FREE PASS.

3. GIVE THEM A RANGE OF MONTHLY DUES, 25 to 35 PER MONTH, PRICE WON'T EVEN BE AN ISSUE. WOULD TODAY BE GOOD OR WOULD TOMORROW BE BETTER?

Chapter 27

PROSPECTING

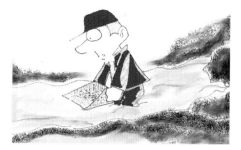

Joe Locke lived in England and like his father before him he did very well with his business. He was a locksmith, and he owned a business selling locks and keys. At the age of 60, he decided it would be time for him to retire. He had prepared for this day for a long time, and he was very happy with his nest egg. He was also happy with his prosperous business and the manner in which it allowed him to provide for his family. As he prepared to close his lock shop, his sons approached him with a question. The oldest son said, "Dad, we always thought that when you decided to retire that we would take over your lock and key business." Joe Locke had taught the boys everything about the lock shop: how to open a lock, how to make keys and how to deal with customers. They were always around. So why was Joe so confused? Suddenly it came to him. When Joe first started his lock and key business he was well schooled in his locksmith trade. He knew everything when it came to the technical aspect of locks and keys.

Perplexed with his reluctance to accept his sons' proposal; his thoughts sunk deeper into his first days as a locksmith. He remembered all of his knowledge of the locksmith trade when he first began. He remembered that even with his knowledge during the first 10 years of the operation he was very poor. Why was he struggling day in and day out? Why was it so hard to make ends meet and why were those first 10 years so difficult? Then it suddenly came to him. He had finally realized that his struggles never came from working with the locks and keys. He realized his challenges were getting more business and getting more people to buy his service.

Happy that he discovered the root of his anguish, he called the boys to a meeting. Joe had decided that he would turn over the lock shop to his sons. The boys were very pleased with his decision and had many new ideas on how to create a successful operation. Joe replied by saying, "Not so fast. There is one condition or requirement. Running your own business is not as easy as it looks. Along with my business I am giving you my name and reputation. In order for me to hand over the business, you must first prove to me that you are capable of handling the highs and lows of this difficult trade." The boys responded by saying, "No problem father, just give us the test."

The test would be a simple one. The oldest son Joe, Jr. would be in charge of the locks and John, the younger son, would be in charge of the keys. Joe, Jr. always seemed to have more of a knack for the technical aspects of fixing the locks and opening doors as John always had more skill when it came to making the keys. Both were ambitious and competitive. They put an ad in the local newspaper and an ad in the local yellow pages. Business started slow but it gradually began to roll in. One of the conditions of their fathers test would be to report back with any discoveries or shortcomings. After a week, both the boys had reported that business had been extremely slow. They also reported that based on the amount of income that was coming in, the lock and key business seemed to be less lucrative than they had originally thought. John, the younger son, decided that on the following day he would go to a busy franchised lock company and study the manner in which they operated their successful business. John immediately noticed that the locksmiths were not as technically advanced as their father. Not only was their technique lacking but the qualities of goods were not up to the standards of their father. "Why was their business so successful? Why were they making so much money," wondered John. John's father had always taught him to look at what people do right and learn from that. John realized that the **key** to the business was not the trade itself. It was the manner in which the business marketed and sold their products.

John reported his findings back to his father and his brother. His father replied by saying that it is good to try new things and if they were so successful, they must have been doing something right. Joe, Jr. responded by saying, "I make the best locks in the land and if I keep doing that, the business will eventually come." John on the other hand was eager to put some of these new techniques into place.

John's first idea was to ask anyone that he had done a lock for if they had any friends or family that were interested or had a need to make keys. (It was amazing how many referrals he received.) He also asked all of his customers if they were interested in having any of the other locks in the house replaced or if they were interested in having a second key made so they would never have this happen again. (Since this problem caused some inconvenience most of John's customers took him up on the offer to have all the keys duplicated.) John gave one free coupon to every customer saying that if you ever lost a key after the initial work was done, the key would be replaced for free. (John also put a little sticker right above the lock that had a phone number for his business.)

These three habits John used with every customer. After a couple of months, Joe Locke called his sons to a meeting to talk about the takeover of the lock and key business. Joe had made a decision based on his sons' performance that he would be turning over the lock and key business. He also asked the boys to submit a report of their progress. Joe discovered that both sons had created a high-quality product. Both sons worked hard, so why was John's business bringing in three times the income of Joe, Jr? Looking at the numbers, Joe Locke had put together a business plan based on John's new inventions. The quality would remain of the highest standards and the business marketing and referrals would be used to operate the already successful business. Joe felt comfortable that his name was in good hands and, not only would he be creating a legacy, but his sons would be successful in achieving financial stability.

The *key* to this chapter and the moral to the story are the same. If you are in business you must have the ability to recruit new clients. In our business you can call it prospecting, generating, getting the door to turn or plane old getting people in. The one thing that has made me successful more than any other thing would be my ability to bring in new business. If you have a terrible closing ratio and you are able to generate volumes when it comes to getting people in the door, you will find a way to be successful.

For Example:

	Yoga counselor No. 1	Yoga counselor No. 2
Opportunities	10	4
Closed deals	6	4
Closing %	60%	100%

Which yoga counselor would you rather be? If each yoga counselor works 300 days per year, the number comes out to the following:

Yoga counselor No. 1= 1,800 deals

Yoga counselor No. 2= 1,200 deals

$50 commission per deal = No. 1 (90, OOO) per year.

$50 commission per deal = No. 2 (70, OOO) per year.

Wow!

This may be shocking but the truth lies in the numbers. Your prospecting habits must be consistent and you may use a plethora of avenues to accomplish this goal. The ones I will give you have made a lot of people rich and have been proven to grow the greatest of company's. "Some of the proven techniques that have worked for me."

Hand Out Passes

The definition of insanity is doing the same thing over and over and expecting a different result.

It is true that every hour members are using our studios, each person has a potential member to offer. No one will argue that, without a doubt, referrals are one of the most valuable sources of new business in our industry. Just as true is the fact that we are not taking advantage of this valuable resource. One of the best ways to approach a member is to offer a guest pass. Again you must adopt the philosophy of "you must give before you ask to receive." If you set aside 20 minutes a day to hand out passes you will find that your hard work will begin to pay off.

Step One

Go out on the floor and tell the members to stop by and see you before they leave. Tell them that you just received some free memberships. "Give before you ask to receive."

Step Two

Make sure your passes are prepared. You must have your initials on the pass and be sure to include an expiration date that ends on closeout.

Step Three

One technique that works well is using a carbon pass that has an area for the name and number of the recipient. That way you can call and confirm the appointment.

Step Four

Just before they are ready to leave your desk, ask them if they have taken advantage of the VIP guest policy. This program is a reward that offers one month for free for every member that you refer to the studio. It is important to get an army of members that are interested in helping you. Remember to take care of these people. They should be the first to receive promotional products like T-shirts or water bottles. Things like these go a long way in the hearts of your members.

Step Five

I staple three passes onto every membership that goes out; this seems to be the best return for my work. I also tell the new member about the VIP guest policy. New members are usually excited about joining the gym so they will tell most of their friends about the passes in the first couple of days.

Step Six

You can also hand out passes in front of stores, schools, restaurants, festivals and in parking lots. It is important not to leave a stack of passes on the counter of a business. The owner will just through them in the garbage. Do your pass distributing daily and make a habit of it. You will get better with time and the new members will start to flow in.

Lead Boxes or Contest Boxes

Many studios have built their business on the lead box and a telephone. This is not my favorite way of getting new business but it is an effective one. Be sure to have the business owner protect your box and keep you informed of the status. It is important to keep your boxes well maintained, clean and stocked.

Since I do not use the old system of lead boxes, I still believe in tracking the success of my contest promotions. You can track the success of your promotion, the quality of the leads, your relationship with the business or even the dates and times of successful promotions. Most companies are still using the old system of lead boxes. They put a box on the counter of a store or retail business. They use it as a trade with business owners who can receive a free membership as long as the box remains there. People fill out entry forms for your studio in hopes to win a one-year membership. As the box fills up, the yoga counselor that set the deal checks the entries and calls the people who have entered. I feel this technique gives our business a bad reputation. Most of the boxes end up not getting tracked or not even getting checked, and the business owners usually just throw them away. I have come up with a highly effective way to utilize the lead boxes. You simply go to a high-traffic location (a supermarket, McDonald's, 7-11, *etc.*) with a lead box and have a contest right then and there.

For example, find a busy nightclub, and you get one or two salespeople at the front door, and everyone who comes in gets to enter in the contest. The contest may say, "Win a trip to Hawaii," which you can get for something like a $100. As the 500 guests come through the door, you let them know in one hour we will be giving away several prizes. In one hour, you can give away workout bags, bottles, T-shirts or free passes to workout in the gym. You also tell people that the Hawaii give-away will be held in the studio on the 31st of the month. You will have to be present to win, and on that day, you will get one more entry into the contest. Also, if you join the studio, you will get five entries into the contest. And, remember to tell them that not a lot of people show up, so they will have a good chance to win. After the drawing, you go back to the studio, and have 500 leads to call to offer two-week passes or set appointments for closeout for the Hawaii giveaway. I use this lead box technique about four times a month. I can usually get 300 to 500 people that are non-members to show up for the end of month closeout sale. When they are in the studio and in an excited mood, our job is made that much easier.

Buddy Referrals

See chapter on Buddy Referrals!

Floor Referrals

Every hour we have hundreds of members using our studios, each with a potential member to offer. No one will argue that without a doubt referrals are the most valuable source of new business in our industry. Just as true is the fact that we are not taking advantage of this valuable resource. One of the main reasons that we fail to get referrals is because of guilty feelings about "bothering" the members. The key to overcoming this feeling is to adopt the philosophy of "you must give before you ask to receive."

Step One

Go through old magazines and cut out articles on yoga and nutrition. After a few hours you will have articles on different body parts, diet and nutrition, injuries, weight loss and more. You should then make copies of these articles and create files for them in your desk.

Step Two

Go out on the workout floor carrying your clipboard and look for members that you can help. Suggest that they stop by your desk before they leave to pick up an article that you think they would be interested in. Build a rapport with the member and ask them to page you if you are not at your desk when they are leaving the studio.

Step Three

Give one of the prepared articles to the member as they are leaving. Be sure to give them an article that contains subject matter that they are sure to have an interest in. Tell the member that you chose this article based on the type of workout that you noticed they were on, or that is based upon what they shared with you about their goals.

Step Four

Just before they are ready to leave your desk, ask them if they have taken advantage of the current promotion in which members are allowed to name three friends to extend an invitation to the studio for a free week. Explain to the member that you must give a certain number of these VIP guest passes, and you would appreciate if they could think of three friends or relatives that may want a free mini-membership. Of course, you always try to get the names and telephone numbers that day, but if they say they will bring names in with them on their next workout, tell them "that would be great, I really appreciate it!" Be sure to give the member a referral form to bring back on their next visit. Also, remember to get the members name and telephone number.

Step Five

Call the member the next day to see if they enjoyed the article. Also, let the member know that you have another article that you want to give them on their next visit. Ask the member when they plan to be in next and remind them not to forget the list of people for the VIP passes.

Business Referrals

Speaking at local employee meetings and organized groups such as Kiwanis, Rotary, Garden, *etc.* is a great way to generate new members.

Step One

Get a copy of the local Chamber of Commerce member's brochure.

Step Two

Prepare a 10-minute speech on the benefits of exercise and good nutrition.

Step Three

Prepare a proposal memo that can be faxed to area groups and businesses offering your services for meetings, luncheons and other group gatherings. Be sure to include your telephone number.

Step Four

Fax your proposal to the different businesses and groups surrounding your studio's location and follow up with a telephone call to verify that it was received. Receive a contact name of who is responsible for putting the meetings together. Contact that person to discuss your proposal. Once they confirm interest, set up the time and place.

Step Five

Bring a T-shirt to the event and a few one-month memberships to give away in a drawing. Allow everyone who attends a chance to enter the drawing before you start your speech. During your speech make sure that you cover all the benefits that your studio has to offer them. They will most likely have questions, so make sure you ask when you finish your segment. It is also a good idea to bring along your business cards to hand out to everyone who attends. Have someone in the crowd complete the drawing for the prizes to be won.

Missed Guests

Ah, missed guest! This would cover all of the guests that have filled out guest yoga profiles. Each and every member that takes a tour of our facility should be tracked. Whether it be in a binder, on a guest yoga profile or in the computer, these missed guests can be a great source of new members.

Step One

Find a list of all the missed guests for the last 30 days. Set aside 30 minutes to one hour to focus on organizing this list.

Step Two

Pay careful attention to the note section of the profile, this may lead to rapport building.

Step Three

Make sure to ask the potential member what their original goals were when they came into the studio in the first place; "This will lead the guest to think for themselves" and ponder why they were so excited about joining.

Step four

For Example:

No. 1: *Hi, is Mary there?* This is Mary! *Mary, this is Mary calling from No. 1 Yoga, and I was just calling to see how every thing was going with your yoga goal.* Oh! I never joined the gym! *Well the reason I called you was to ask a very simple question. What was your goal when you came down to the center.* Well I wanted to lose some weight! *Mary why don't you come down to the studio today and we can get you started on a pass! What works best for you morning or evening?*

TI and Guest Register

Old TIs and guest registers are usually causing a fire hazard in your file cabinet or cupboard. Give me a telephone and a stack of old guest registers, and I can make a great living. When calling back old guest registers and TI's be sure to make notes and if they have an address you can certainly send a postcard.

Step One

When I first started at a gym as a young manager, one of the ways that I improved my personal sales would be to call all of the missed guest registers and TI's. I would simply leave a message on their machine.

Step Two

I would even go though the old member lists. Every day, I would call at least 100 people. *"Hi, this is Ron. I am the new manager from Number One Yoga, as a new manager, I just want to introduce myself. If you have any questions or friends you want to bring to our gym, call me and I will take care of them personally. Also, if you have any problems or concerns my door is always open."* Ten people a day would come in to greet me and ask how much it will cost to upgrade or sign up their friends. One short message on an answering machine can make members happy, feel important or even refer family members. Our members bring in more sales than anything else. So get in touch with your members.

Step Three

Call your old TI's and say you are calling from the customer service department at No.1 Yoga and you were doing a quality control call. Every person that participates will receive a two-week free membership.

Front Desk Computer

The front desk computer can be a great way to increase your personal sales. If your check-in system is like mine, you can see updated information pertaining to every member. The following information may be of use: what kind of membership, when it will expire, a picture, family add-on information and more. If I were a new yoga counselor, I would simply stand in front of the computer and remind every member to bring their card. You will be surprised how many members owe money or find that those who are on contracts will expire soon. With a few clicks, the computer can also print out a list of soon-expiring members. A large percentage of your members may be on short-term or pre-paid memberships that may be upgraded or renewed. It is very simple.

Step One

Ask all the check-ins if they are enjoying their workouts and if the studio is helping them accomplish their goals.

Step Two

Ask all the check-ins if they have tried the other locations in the area and if they are interested in upgrading to use other facilities or services.

Step Three

Ask how the one-on-one yoga or nutrition classes are going and if they are interested in trying one for free.

Step Four

Meeting and greeting every member at the front desk will drastically improve your referral business. This is just good customer service. Be sure to use their first name and always smile. This is a great way to get in good with your membership base.

Our Staff

We have hundreds of employees, but only a small percentage of them are allowed to sell memberships. However, every yoga instructor, front-desk employee or personal instructor will have friends willing to join the studio. You can give a staff member that brings friends into join the studio something in return. You should be the town mayor. Work a deal with everyone in the studio to give their referrals to you. You must ABC, Always Be Closing. There are so many ways to make money. You simply go out and use the tools that have been given to you. Networking, prospecting and building rapport with the staff will increase sales tremendously.

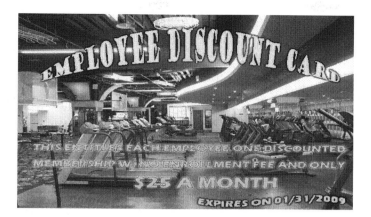

Step one

You might offer a contest to the employees. The employee who has the most guest passes with their initials can win a trip or a dinner (use trade outs).

Step two

Offer to split commission with the employee that brings in a new yoga member.

Step three

Offer a paid day off to the top referral employee. This may be all they need to start sending new members your way. I have worked many days for my staff members that have helped me win sales contests.

Step four

Offer studio services, such as tanning or one-on-one yoga, even a free membership could be the answer.

Door Hangers

A person may not open every piece of mail, but they will always open their door.

Step One

Design and create a door hanger that will get a person's attention at a first glance. Preferably the door hanger should have a "hot" photo or a "free" offer of some type. Use as few words as possible and bold type for easy reading. It is also smart to state "limited time offer." Be sure to include your address and telephone number. (The door hanger must go through the appropriate approval process.)

Step Two

Inquire on how to purchase or receive a local address directory. This directory will list all residents that have a listed telephone number by street address. Once you have possession of this directory, it is only a matter of time before your sales increase drastically.

Step Three

Be sure to put your name on each of the door hangers that you distribute. Some prefer to staple a business card to each door hanger.

Step Four

Decide on the amount of door hangers that you are to distribute each week. Some counselors prefer to hit the streets for one or two hours per day, while others prefer to go out every other day. A realistic goal would be to distribute 20 to 50 hangers per day. Keep a detailed list of every address that you delivered a hanger.

Step Five

Once you have achieved your distribution goal, it's time to turn your hard work into sales. Using your directory; call every household that you left a door hanger.

Sample Telephone Script:

Hi, my name is _____ with Number One Yoga. I wanted to call to confirm that you received the free membership offer that we delivered to your home? Did you receive it? Great! Well, I would like to answer any questions that you might have about the studio and also explain some of the exciting details about the free membership you've been chosen to receive.

New Residents

Every month, at least 100 new residents move to within five miles of your studio. These residents are basically not approached until they decide to seek a local yoga center to join. Why wait for them to find us? Let's introduce ourselves.

Step One

Make a list of all local apartment complexes and residential brokers.

Step Two

Create a welcome gift that includes a one-month membership and a buddy gift. (Pass length and buddy gifts may vary.)

Step Three

Contact each apartment manager and real estate office manager to explain the Number One Yoga "Welcome Package" program. Also explain about our VIP Month-to-Month Free program (pass length may vary by division) that we offer to all managers who participate in the program.

Step Four

Bring in a sample "Welcome Package" for display at each location that you have arranged to participate in the program. Be sure to give the manager plenty of guest passes, in addition to their VIP membership pass to your location.

Step Five

Call each location weekly to receive the names and numbers of the past weeks' new homebuyers or renters. Understand that sometimes it takes a few days to get their telephone connected. The rest is easy!

Corporate Draws

Step One

Locate all potential businesses in your area including corporate centers, shopping centers, strip malls and food courts.

Step Two

Assign specific areas to each counselor to avoid duplication in certain centers. Each counselor can then establish business relationships with the existing businesses in each center.

Step Three

The counselor should designate a few hours in order to properly "work" the specified area for the day. The only materials you need are pens and lead slips. Since there is potential for setting up lead boxes in some locations, a supply of these would be appropriate.

Step Four

Authorization for office complexes and shopping malls will be necessary if not already established. In most business complexes there is no one individual to approve this type of solicitation. If you are asked to stop by a security guard do so immediately. In shopping malls try to use established relationships with the malls in your area. If you do not have an existing relationship with a particular mall, proceed as if you had permission until someone tells you otherwise. At this point, go to the mall manager's office and express your apologies and ask them for the proper way to solicit.

Step Five

Obtain leads on a person-to-person basis.

Sample Script:

Hi, my name is _____ with Number One Yoga. I am giving away two, three-month memberships. Are you currently a member with us? "No" Great! Place your name on this entry form and I will enter you in the drawing. The winner will be drawn at 9 a.m. tomorrow morning and will be notified by noon. Thank you and good luck!

Business of the Week

Step One

Call or visit retail merchants in your area and tell them you are representing Number One Yoga and would like to tell them about our Cross-Promotion Program.

Step Two

Inform the manager/owner of the benefits that the studio can provide to companies that partake in this program.

Step Three

Tell them that all we would like in return is to display our advertising and promotional boxes at their place of business. Ask when they would like to be scheduled as the "Business of the Week."

Step Four

Fill out the Business of the Week request form and place lead box in retail outlet.

Step Five

Register the location on the lead box section of your daily planner and pick up the leads in seven days.

Local Colleges Promotion

Step One

Visit all of the local colleges and read all local newspapers and advertisements to see what upcoming events are scheduled for them. It is vital that you get permission to be on any college campus.

Step Two

Contact the local college student marketing departments or the associated student body departments.

Step Three

When speaking with the college representative, explain that you would like to help support their next event by setting up a promotional table to giveaway free short-term memberships plus have a drawing for T-shirts, water bottles and more. Most local colleges have events scheduled throughout the school year. However, if they don't, recommend that they have a health fair on campus consisting of free short-term memberships to the yoga center as well as hosting blood pressure checks, body fat testing and more.

Sample script:

"Hello_____, my name is _____. I'm with Number One Yoga. We are currently conducting promotions with local colleges like yours where we come out to the campus and give all the students free short-term memberships, plus a chance to enter to win a six month membership, T-shirts, water bottles and more. This promotion would be done courtesy of the (ASB, student marketing or whoever you are working with). We are scheduling our promotions now and would like to know if the first or second week of this month would be good for you, and how many free short term memberships do you think you would need."

Step Four

Meet with studio management to make sure you have the supplies that are needed.

Table	One week and one visit guest passes
Wheel of Fortune	Water bottles
Lead slips	T-shirts
Pencils	Number One Yoga banner
	Approved spin and win signage

Step Five

Arrive to the event early to set up. Make sure that your banner is placed professionally and in a highly visible location. Come fully prepared. If the promotion goes well, you can regularly attend their events and have a continuous lead source.

Grocery Store Promotion

A well planned grocery store promotion has always proven to be very successful. Major grocery stores have great traffic, resulting in high volume lead generation within a short period of time.

Step One

Scope your studio's territory for the large grocery store chains.

Step Two

Contact the store's general manager. Explain the benefits and the overall set up of the promotion and that you will be offering free body fat testing and will be giving away short-term memberships, T-shirts and water bottles. Ask for a position inside the store as it is a better environment for people to stop and be presented. If not inside, the front of the store can be successful. The best days to set up the promotion are; Wednesdays and Saturdays, the 1st and the 15th, and the days before any holidays. These days generally have very high traffic.

Step Three

A trade or purchase of a $100 store gift certificate can double and even triple your lead generation totals. When you purchase the gift certificate, have your approved promotional sign highlight the $100 giveaway. On a holiday promotion and holiday weekends, tie in your giveaway to that specific holiday. For example, the promotion can say, "Win a Thanksgiving Gift Certificate for $100."

Step Four

You may want to offer the general manager a VIP membership so he or she can enjoy the benefits of the yoga center. (Pass length may very by division.)

Step Five

In addition to the display in the health isle, (or instead of), get cooperation from the cashiers and have a friendly competition. Set up a small acrylic lead box at each check stand so customers can enter the drawing for the shopping spree, memberships or *any* vendor provided prizes. Have a drawing each day and post the winners names on a display board. Each cashier has a locked acrylic lead box assigned to them. The cashier with the most entries wins. A large acrylic lead box can be displayed at the check out counter for a two-week or one-month drawing.

Sample Script to Use for the General Manager:

"Hello (store manager), this is (your name) from Number One Yoga. We are currently performing outside promotions with major grocery stores such as yours. The promotion works well to introduce our community and you benefit by giving all your staff and customers free short-term memberships as well as other gifts such as T-shirts, water bottles, free body fat testing or a chance to win a $100 gift certificate. This promotion costs you nothing to put on, as we handle everything. Now (store manager), we could set up inside your store by the health food aisle on Wednesday morning or Saturday morning, which would be better for you?"

Make sure that you have the following items on the day of the promotion:

Table	One week/ one visit guest passes
Wheel of fortune	Water bottles
Lead Slips	T-shirts
Pencils	Number One Yoga Banner
	Approved spin and win signage

This promotion can also be accomplished with sporting good stores, pharmacies and more.

Movie Theater Promotion

Theaters are a viable source to generate leads, especially on a Friday or Saturday night.

Step One

Obtain a list of all of the local movie theaters in your area. Establish contact with the theater manager and offer them a mutually beneficial promotional relationship.

Step Two

Offer the manager a free short-term membership so he/she can enjoy the benefits of Number One Yoga. Explain how, on an ongoing basis, Number One Yoga can offer the theaters an opportunity to promote their latest movie releases to our members by displaying a poster or display at Number One Yoga. The poster should inform our members of the movie and that anyone with a Number One Yoga membership can show their card at the box office and get a free popcorn. Reciprocally, anyone showing their ticket stub at Number One Yoga will receive a short-term membership. A poster at the theater indicating this should be displayed prominently with a nice acrylic lead box nearby so they may enter and win memberships, movie tickets and more.

Step Three

Now that you've established a relationship with the theater, periodically (preferably on Friday or Saturday nights) bring the Wheel of Yoga to the theater and set it up in the lobby. The theater can usually give you prizes for the wheel such as movie tickets, posters, concessions, coupons and more. If it is possible, have at least two people staff the promotion, have one person man the wheel and the other person work outside with the people in line. The people in line need something to do during their long wait. They can fill out the entry slip and do the spin and win when they get inside. The grand prize of a six-month membership should be given away at the end of the night.

Sample script:

"Hi, this is (your name), from Number One Yoga located at (address). We would like to promote your theater and movie releases to our members. In addition, we would like to offer anyone with your theater ticket stub a free short-term membership to Number One Yoga. Would you be interested in promoting your theater to our members in this theater? We can also give out prizes to your guests. Will this Friday and Saturday be okay with you to begin this promotion?"

Step Four

Meet with your general manager and front desk manager to gather up the supplies needed prior to the promotion:

Table	Water bottles
Wheel of fortune	T-shirts
Lead slips	Number One Yoga banner
Pencils	Approved spin and signage

One week and one visit guest passes

Step Five

Arrive early to set up and come prepared. Promotions with movie theaters can be lucrative and can bring in hundreds of leads per night, if done correctly.

Member Appreciation Day

"Member Appreciation Day" is a great event to plan for a power day of leads, appointments and gross.

Step One

Contact vendors for food, entertainment and free samples. Offer free T-shirts or water bottles for referrals or enrollments. Trade or buy a "must be present to win" prize. Promote your Member Appreciation Day with announcements and flyers.

Step Two

Have your one-on-one yoga department supply free blood pressure testing, body fat testing and complimentary one-on-one yoga sessions.

Step Three

Have each counselor promote guests for the day. For example, "(Mr. Member), this Thursday is our Member Appreciation Day. We will be having free blood pressure checks, body fat testing, food and entertainment. I just need to pre-register your friends and coworkers who will be attending with you this Thursday. (Get names and numbers of the referrals). "Great, we'll invite them for this Thursday as your guests for Member Appreciation Day. If they enjoy the studio and do enroll you'll receive _____."

Step Four

Have the entire staff set appointments for the referrals for your Member Appreciation Day. Appointments script example follows: "Mr. Referral, this is (your name) at Number One Yoga. Mr. Member gave us your name and number and asked that we invite you in as his/her guest this Thursday for Member Appreciation Day. You'll receive a free short-term membership, free blood pressure and body fat testing plus food and entertainment. Mr. Referral, what type of results would you like to get from a yoga program? *Response*, great, we can show you an exercise program that will help you accomplish those goals. We have (explain facilities)." Confirm appointment time, location and have them write down your telephone number and your name. (If Mr. Referral cannot book for the Member Appreciation Day, book within 48 hours.)

Step Five

Member Appreciation Day checklist:

1. Create and print with proper approval invitations and flyers announcing your Member Appreciation Day party.

2. Distribute invitations and flyers out to local businesses, Chamber of Commerce mixers and other businesses.

3. Have the staff remind the local businesses and members about the party.

4. Call all the pre-registered guests to remind them about the party.

5. Make announcements about the party on the PA system.

6. Have a food supply of buddy gifts available for the party.

7. Contact local restaurants and do a trade for food and beverages.

8. Work with your yoga supervisor to make sure they have a demonstration class planned.

9. Work with your One-on-one yoga Department to make sure they are set up to conduct body fat testing, blood pressure checks, complimentary one-on-one yoga training.

10. Schedule extra floor instructors for guest tours.

11. Schedule extra child care employees and offer free child care for the day.

Health Fair and Marathon Promotion

This promotion will create leads, community exposure and a festive atmosphere for your current and potential members.

Step One

Set up a health fair and yoga or cardio equipment marathon in your studio by selling booth space in your facility for the day of the event. A local merchant (doctors, chiropractors, massage therapists, nutrition experts, beauticians, *etc.*) will normally pay up to $500 if you allow them to advertise in your studio for a month and sell product and promote their business the day of the event. If you can get 10 to 15 participants you now have enough money to fund the promotion. These booths should cover the cost of internal and external flyers, and advertising on radio and newspapers. The media will really get behind the event if it involves a charity or nonprofit group, and you give all of the proceeds to the charity. Many of these large nonprofit groups have the resources and have been trained on how to put on events that create exposure and donations.

Step Two

In addition to the health fair booth fees, you can also set up a yoga marathon with the nonprofit group to create proceeds to cover expenses and generate donations for the charity. Have your staff and the charity go door to door, and business to business getting pledges for the amount of minutes or hours that they will be doing yoga (each sponsor will get a free short-term membership in addition to a tax deduction). At the same time, they can collect leads, sell rate reservations and hand out flyers. You can also set up card table booth space in malls and supermarkets (high traffic areas) to promote the event. In addition to promoting outside, you should be promoting inside your studio as well.

Step Three

Have a person in charge of going to local merchants, the media and large corporations for donations or trade outs of their product to be used for the event such as food, a DJ, radio live remote, decorations, prizes and more.

Step Four

Now that you have set up the marketing and promotion of the health fair and marathon you need to set up the product and justification for the fair. You need to have cholesterol testing, body compositions, blood pressure testing and more. If you can get the cholesterol testing donated, great, if not, charge a small fee to cover the cost. A well-known supermarket once promoted this with a charity backing them and it became a huge success with more than 4,000 people showing up one Saturday each paying $10 for the testing. You should be able to attract 250 to 500 new guests throughout the month.

Step Five

The day of the event should run smoothly. If planned, promoted and carried out correctly, the nonprofit organization will see great potential (pledges, donations and the $5 rate reservations) and will really get behind the promotion with their power and expertise. Make sure that you have greeters, additional staff for tours, full sales staff, free child care for guests and special yoga classes (which you have promoted in your advertisements), plenty of food and entertainment, as well as a festive, well decorated, grand opening atmosphere. If promoted effectively, inside and outside of the studio, you can create added walk-ins, and telephone inquiries into the studio. This will add to the donations and good will.

Chapter 28

HOW TO HANDLE

PASSES

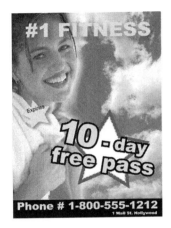

Most yoga centers still use the pass as their No.1 source of advertising. I see many salespeople who are afraid to take a guest with a pass because they are afraid they will not be able to overcome the "*I want to try it first*" objection. I agree it is harder to sign somebody up that has a pass, rather than a person simply coming in to the studio to join. On the other hand, I do feel that if you have been properly trained and are not afraid to take passes, you can substantially increase your paycheck. The overall census of new yoga center sales manuals advised to give them their passes and let them try it and sign them up after. I disagree, my studio statistics show that 60 percent of all the people that used passes never used the studio after the day the pass was given. This means, that out of 10 people that use their passes, you will only have four guests that will come back after the pass to become members; even if you have a 100 percent closing ratio. You will only have a 40 percent closing ratio. I do not know of anyone who can close 10 out of 10 of these types of guests.

There are also studios that give the pass right away and try to get the guest to trade it back in on a discounted membership. I feel the best way to help people accomplish their goals is to sign them up before they try the studio. Why give someone 10 days to get sore or hurt themselves when they have long-term goals in mind? They are looking for long-term results, and we are giving them a short-term membership. To me, that does not make sense. I feel that if the person is not happy with our studio, they should be entitled to a refund. Remember, people wake up every morning with the best intentions to change their lives, *"Today I am going to start saving money. Today I am going to quit smoking. Today I am going to eat right. Today I am going to start exercising."* By noon, our brain has tricked our body into putting everything off until the next day. These tricks that our minds play on our body are similar to a smokers thought process. Procrastination is a disease that prevents us from accomplishing goals in life. Stop setting yourself up for failure. I hate to quote Nike, but the only way to accomplish anything in this life is to *"just do it."* You cannot think about it, you cannot talk about it, you have to just start. Please feel free to use the steps outlined in the chapter on closing.

Chapter 29

SALES PRESENTATION CHECKLIST

The sales manager or general manager should always have a sales presentation checklist. This list does not need to be used all the time but whenever you feel like your sales percentage is going down, you can refer back to this list to help you establish a reason. This list can also work for you personally, as you can refer to it for areas of weaknesses. It is a checklist of questions for random members or "company shoppers" to fill out to rate the overall sale.

For Example:

- Did the front desk person greet me quickly and friendly?
- Did the front desk person appear well groomed and make good eye contact?
- Did the staff eat or chew gum during the tour?
- Did the front desk person ask me to fill out the guest profile?
- Did the yoga counselor approach the guest in a timely manner?
- Did the yoga counselor appear well-groomed and friendly?
- Did the yoga counselor use the introduction?
- Did the yoga counselor fill out the back of the guest profile and seem generally concerned with your goal?
- Did they take you on a tour of the facility?

- Did they seem knowledgeable about the studio and answer all of your questions?

- Did they ask you for your commitment of joining the studio today?

- Did they show you the different membership options or offer other services such as one-on-one yoga?

- Did the yoga counselor make several attempts to get you started on a membership?

- Did you feel the yoga counselor was overly aggressive?

- Did the yoga counselor bring another staff member into the presentation?

- Did the yoga counselor give you a pass or make an appointment to see you on a later date?

- Was the studio clean?

- Did the other staff members seem to be working?

- If you joined, did the yoga counselor make an appointment for the first work out or give you passes for friends or family?

This checklist can be used for mystery shoppers or for the manager to critique the yoga counselor's performance. It is a tool that can be used to illustrate what are the strong points and the weak points of your studio. It allows for a non-biased assessment of your studio, asking the major questions that you, as a manger or yoga counselor, want to know the answers to. I do not use this checklist to punish salespeople or myself.

It only outlines areas that can be improved on or areas that have been missed out altogether. I use the result of these periodical checklists to give me a fresh view of what we, as a studio, need to work on. It allows me to see and hear what our members think about our studio.

Chapter 30

FREE ONE-ON-ONE YOGA

In our studios, we have a program called "Quick Results"; it is the feeder program for our one-on-one yoga revenue. It is also a yoga orientation to help our members have some general knowledge of exercise. These programs vary from studio to studio, but a good yoga introduction especially to a person on a pass can be the difference of converting free passes into memberships. Our studio gives two sessions of one-on-one yoga at no cost, especially if the guest shows some interests or lack of knowledge in exercise. We will use our one-on-one yoga presentation to recommend on-going one-on-one programs.

I truly believe that the members involved in one-on-one yoga refer the most people to our studios and are the most successful members in terms of results. Everyone who purchases a membership or gets a pass should get the quick results program. At the end of the quick results program, they should be brought to the sales department along with the instructors to talk about how their orientation went, find out which vitamins they need and if they are interested in on-going one-on-one sessions. The more people that go through this program, the more training sales your studio will have.

Chapter 31

HOW TO INTERACT WITH

THE STAFF

S taff interaction is an overlooked yet vital aspect of our business. Many sales managers and yoga consultants fail to lay down the groundwork, to interact well with others. Loving your job or dreading the thought of even showing up to work could all depend on how well you work with your surrounding staff. Since we are in a commission driven business, salespeople can become competitive. And at times will even cross the line of stealing or "sharking" sales. The way to handle these problems is quickly, privately and usually through your manager. Problems that are not handled immediately can fester into much larger problems that can affect the entire studio. Staff members that will allow the other sales counselors to take hard earned commission will most certainly become a target of lost income. Make sure that you are clear on all the rules when it comes to splitting commissions, "be-back appointments", appointments in the MAB, telephone inquiries or "ask-fors." I will just give a little example of how our studio handles commissions. If a yoga counselor has an appointment, it must be in their planner or in the MAB. If it is not, it is not an appointment. That appointment must be within 24 hours of the day it is written in the book, (same day, day before, day after). If another person takes your appointment, it is a split. If you have a person come back to the studio, and it is not in the MAB. And they do not ask for you, it is not yours. If a person comes into the studio and asks for you, that is your "ask-for" or appointment.

If you are with a walk-in, you will receive half. If a person on your pass joins the studio, and they don't join with you, and you don't have an appointment, you will get nothing. (You should have closed them when you had the chance.) Renewals belong to the person that sells them, not to the person who signs them up originally. (If you did a good job on your post-sale, nobody would renew with anyone but you.) Assistant mangers, general managers or future managers should be doing the TO's. TO's should never be split. New salespeople will not TO if you take half of their deals. Lastly passes should have the counselor's name on them, if not, they are ups.

These are just some of the rules we run at our studios. We have used these rules for years, and they work very well. Remember, what comes around goes around. And if you are not consistent, that is where you will run into problems. Again, remember, to handle your issues immediately and consistently. You may even consider posting the rules, so that everybody is clear. In one of the studios I worked in, the manager had the sales staffs vote on each rule. He then posted the rules on the wall, and we never had a problem.

The most important relationship you can have will be with your front desk staff, as they are the first contact. They can control your paycheck.

Different studios run different rotations. I found that in a majority of studios the managers will give the most ups to the best closer or the top grosser, other studios run an up's list. The top grosser from the previous day is first on the list. Other studios require a certain amount of appointments to be on rotation. Whichever one of these systems your studio uses, you want to make sure that you are on this list or rotation. Get on it and stay on it. The yoga business can sometimes be considered too lackadaisical of an environment to be considered work, and people tend to get lazy. Remember, winning is a habit, and losing is a habit. If you show up to work at ten o'clock, read the newspaper and go get a cup of coffee, and at eleven o'clock take a guest, by noon you are at an hour lunch, come back at one and have a training meeting, talk to the other salespeople for an hour, go workout, then go to dinner, you can see it will be very difficult to be a top producer. And it can also make for low sales and lack of promotions. I have a to-do list that I consistently follow. I don't hang out with the "fun bunch" until everything on my list is finished. In the chapter on time management, I have put my eight steps for success. The reason it is only eight steps is because I feel that if it is too complicated, it will not get completed. I feel that if each step is done everyday, it will be worth $8,000 on your paycheck. For each step that you fail to complete, subtract $1,000 off of your paycheck.

Negativity is the cancer that ruins your paycheck. Do not get caught up in other people's business. Mom always says, "Mind your own business." Remember, if you have complaints or something negative to say, complaints go up. Complaints don't go level or down, they go up. Keep focused on your business at hand, stay away from the fun bunch and have clear rules of commission. Stay on the ups list and follow your to-do list every single day. By following simple rules of staff interaction, you will truly love your job in the yoga industry.

Mother Teresa of Calcutta quotes

If you are kind, people may accuse you of selfish, ulterior motives:

Be kind anyway.

People are often unreasonable, illogical and self-centered:

Forgive them anyway.

If you are successful, you will win some false friends and some true enemies:

Succeed anyway.

If you are honest and frank, people may cheat you:

Be honest and frank anyway.

What you spend years building, someone may destroy overnight:

Build anyway.

If you find serenity and happiness, they may be jealous:
Be happy anyway.
The good you do today, people will often forget tomorrow:
Do good anyway.
Give the world the best you have, and it may never be enough:
Give the world the best you have anyway
You see, in the final analysis, it is all between you and god:
It was never between you and them anyway.

Mother Teresa of Calcutta!

Chapter 32

A MENTOR

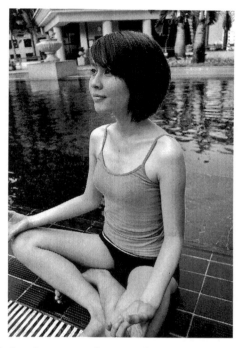

Not everyone starts off with great instincts when it comes to sales, but whatever abilities people have can be nurtured and developed. My first six months as a yoga counselor were very difficult. I felt that I was good with people but I did not have much in the way of natural sales ability. The system that I put together is geared towards people like myself: the 99 percent that are not gifted in sales. I feel that anyone can sell memberships if they have the determination and ability to learn the system. There was no system when I started; it was just me and my mentor. He showed me his methods, he critiqued my weak points, gave me encouragement, TOed for me, helped me understand the rules of the game and showed me the correct way to fill out membership agreements.

I owe most of my early success to my mentor. I probably would not have lasted as a yoga counselor if I would not have had someone like this to help me. What did he gain in return? That is a simple answer. I worked on his team. If he needed to have someone to stay late, or come in early, I was there. If he needed someone to work on Sunday, I was there. When he became a general manager, I followed him to every studio he went. I followed out every task he asked down to the smallest detail. When he became a district manager, he promoted me to general manager. He sent me to whatever studio that was doing poorly. I followed the system and brought the low studios up to being the top studios. This relationship helped our company be more successful, and, in turn, we helped each other become more successful. We made more money, because we worked together. If you do not have a mentor, your road to success may be much slower. Remember, when you work your way to the top, you are going to need loyal people under you.

Mentoring is crucial because you also learn when you teach. We use the word **TEAM**:

Together Everybody Achieves More.

I have mentored hundreds of salespeople and many general managers. If I had an opportunity to operate yoga centers again, most of them would be willing to make a transition to work under my management. This is one of my most valuable assets. I always have the resources to get some of the top managers in the yoga center business. This is only possible because I mentored them. Finding a mentor is simple. If you are a beginning yoga counselor, find the top salesman in your studio, the one with the best reputation and the numbers to go along with it. If you happen to be that top yoga counselor, find yourself a new employee to mentor: somebody like yourself who is looking to absorb what you have to offer. This relationship benefits both the mentor and the understudy because you are working together to hone both of your skills and are working together towards a common goal. You will find that a real bond and loyalty is formed, which can benefit your studio and your sales.

Chapter 33

HOW TO MAKE SIGNS

They call me the "sign guy." I put signs everywhere in the studio, hundreds of them, using bright colors that stand out, with big writing and always with an expiration date. I leave them up two days after the promotion expires. I use words such as final day, hurry, don't miss out, last chance, limited time, special, once in a lifetime and never again. The reason I leave them up after they expire is that it creates a sense of urgency and finality to the promotion. I tell inquiring members that the program has already expired, but if I can get that deal for them, would they want to get started right away. I always put the tape on the four conrners on the back of the signs, so they do not look messy and I put them everywhere.

For Example:

No Enrollment fee!, Family Add-On Prices!, Buy a Year Get a Year Free!, Weekend Sale, 3 Sessions of One-on-one yoga - $99!, Half-Off Supplements Today Only!, 25% off all retail!

If you are not using signs or having sales in the studio, you are missing the boat. Go into any retail business and you will see signs: from grocery stores, 10 for a dollar on oranges, bonus buy on grocery items, to markdown signs at car dealerships, to happy hour specials at a local pub, one dollar happy hour drink and more. Signs motivate sales. For example, I have a furniture store two blocks from my home. They have signs all over the windows that simply say "Going out of Business Sale!" and "Store closes in 30 Days!" This furniture store has been going out of business for 10 years and people are always rushing in to buy merchandise there. All because of the signs and the sense of urgency that it creates within the buyer. Trust me signs work. Let's say that you go into a clothing store and you see that a shirt is marked down from $100 to $20. You look at the tag, and you see the $100 price tag is crossed out and has been re-written with red ink that says $20. I would venture to guess that the shirt never really cost $100 in the first place. It is simply the clothing store using their retail knowledge and sales skills to make people believe they are getting a good deal. If you put two racks of shirts side by side, on one side there is a rack of shirts for $20, on the other side, there is a rack of shirts marked down from $100 to $20. These shirts could look exactly the same, but the marked down shirts will sell 90 percent faster.

My wife walks in the house from a busy day at the shopping mall. She has a big fat smile on her face and has several bags in her hand. I ask her if she went shopping. She says to me, "Look at all the money I saved." I reply to her that she did a great job saving money but "why did you buy another jacket, when you already have one just like it?" Then she says her favorite saying, "I had to, because it was on sale!" She then responds "I bought you a new shirt," and I say, "I already have 20 shirts just like that shirt." She responds by saying 'If you don't want it, can I have it?' Sales are key to continued growth in the yoga center business and signs that display the sale are just as key.

Chapter 34

THE CLOSEOUT

MASTER PLAN

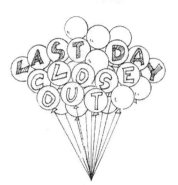

This is something that you should have in your planner. You should always go over starting a couple days before closeout to make sure you are successful. Closeout represents about five days worth of revenue. One bad closeout is equal to five bad days. One good closeout is worth five good days. Be aware of this and make sure that you are set up and ready. Remember, yoga centers are about energy. The best operators are the ones that can create energy, not only among the members and guests, but among the staff. "Macy's white flower day," if you can tell me what a white flower day is, then you are smarter than me. The most successful day in retail sales for many years was a closeout created by Macy's Department Store. It has nothing to do with anything other than a sale and the energy created by it.

Key Elements to Creating a Closeout

All passes will expire that day. All corporate open enrollment periods should be expiring that day. All special pricing will be expiring that day. One hundred "hot colored signs will be up in the studio, announcements are being made every 10 minutes, the telephone is answered in a different way and all schedules are cleared of member problems, one-on-one yoga sessions or nutrition sessions. Closeout is set up for sales only. Post-dated checks or credit cards should all be made for the 15th or the 30th of the month, this creates excitement among the staff. The contest box for the trip give-a-way should be front and center: The most important part about the trip give-a-way is that you have to be present to win and you have to bring a non-member to enter. The two most important elements are the raffle in the evening or throughout the day and several outside vendors coming in to promote their product. This will create a festive atmosphere in your studio. Make sure that all staff is at the studio at 8:00 a.m. and that the studio is decorated by 9:00 a.m. Make sure to have one person scheduled to come in extremely early because there is a whole group of members and guests that like to come in early and you may miss an opportunity. You may be able to upgrade a membership or sell them one-on-one yoga. The person that wants to make the biggest paycheck is probably the person that will be there early.

The Set Up

1. Assign each counselor a job for closeout. An example is making someone in charge of setting up the supplement booth, setting up the outside vendors or making sure the studio is decorated with balloons. Sit down and have a plan for the day. The way you are successful is that you have a plan and that you work the plan.

2. Each counselor should have a 20-appointment goal set. Set this at the beginning of the month. Let members know that the last day of the month is a great day for deals and if they can't make it now to make an appointment for closeout. Make your telephone calls and confirm your passes the day before closeout.

3. Each counselor is required to call 50 current members and 100 missed guests to promote the closeout. Call to let people know what great opportunities will be available on closeout and that any non-member can come into the studio for free. Explain that there is a big party, give-a-ways and great deals.

4. Signs must be up. Counselors should know the promotion, have a plan and confirm deals coming in. The staff schedule for closeout is 8:00 a.m. to 8:00 p.m. Make sure promotional signs are posted everywhere and know what the current promotion is. Have a production meeting to ensure that all staff knows the promotion and what the signs mean.

5. All "balance dues" and "promise to pays" must be collected or scheduled for closeout. Everyone that owes money should be called and told to come in on closeout to pay their balance or they will be sent to collections.

6. Advise the front desk of telephone salutations and start it today. "Thank you for calling _____on our closeout sale, how may I help you?" Promote whatever the special is on the telephone salutation. Attach it to the telephone.

7. One counselor should be working the front desk all day for "flips" and renewals. Make sure that one person is at the desk working check-ins and making sure that every person that walks in is told about the specials. This is a huge source of revenue for the company.

8. Before counselors go home make sure that all appointments are written in the master appointment book.

9. All post dates should be put on the books and make sure to write them down the night before closeout. This way you know exactly how much needs to be made to hit your goal.

10. Fill the hype with each and every employee about the big day that is happening tomorrow. Make sure that everyone knows and understands what closeout is.

11. The front desk should have a retail or sidewalk sale set up and they should handle any food, fashion shows or sidewalk sales. Instructors should be doing orientations, potential sales only and be in charge of supplement or one-on-one yoga seminars in the yoga room. Nutritionists should clear their schedules and be in charge of vitamin seminars or nutrition seminars. Yoga instructors should do a dance seminar

at some point in the evening or a spinning demonstration out in front of the studio.

12. Closeout should not cost the company money. Closeout should be part of the employees job description and the staff gets paid extra commission based on extra sales. All trips, food and vendors should be traded out with the approval of the general manager or regional manager. No trade outs can be used for personal benefits.

On the Day of Closeout

On the day of closeout you should have this list posted in your office and on your planner and you should make sure to do everything on the list.

1. On closeout, have a morning production meeting and motivate everybody. Get them excited. Let everyone know what is riding on the studios performance; let them know where the studio is at and what needs to be done to hit your goals.

2. Get balloons, streamers, and signs up so the studio looks like there is a party going on.

3. Don't deal with any cancellations or customer service issues today. Today is pure production. No negativity is allowed.

4. Do 25 percent off retail and supplements and set up booths for promotion of this. Buy 2 get the 3rd one free or buy 1 and get the 2nd for 50 percent off.

5. Continue over the telephone promoting for the evening.

6. No workouts for employees allowed on closeout.

7. Emphasize pre-paid options. Every deal three, six or 18 months free.

8. Make sure you have something to give-a-way to members. Do trade-outs with businesses to give in a drawing on closeout. This creates a buying atmosphere.

9. Have an afternoon production meeting.

10. Nobody "walks" on closeout. Call your district manager to approve deals.

11. Dress in a different, or new neatly pressed uniform. Appearance and presence are half the battle.

Chapter 35

TIME MANAGEMENT

Time management is an area that is standard in all businesses. Everything from students, to the common housewives, to the CEO must have a structured system that creates good habits. I cannot stress enough the effect time management can have on your success in life. You only have so much time; when the time is up, your life is over. Procrastination takes over, bad habits are formed and we never accomplish things in life because we do not have good time management skills.

One of the owners that I used to work for always told a story about his ditch digging theory. He would say that one of his employees would spend all day digging a ditch. It was a perfect ditch: It was deep, it was long and it was perfectly round. He worked hard all day, and he was happy with his accomplishment. When he was finished, he would come back into the studio and say, "I worked hard all day. I even have blisters on my hands and now I am finally done. Isn't it a beautiful ditch?" And the owner would reply, "That is great, and it is a beautiful ditch. There is only one problem: We don't need a ditch!"

The story is to remind you that your job is to sell memberships and make appointments for memberships. It is important to keep *the main thing the main thing*. Work smart, not hard, and stay focused on the business at hand. If your studio is like mine, you only get paid for sales. Do you realize that if you spend 10 minutes a day saving money, 10 minutes a day learning a foreign language, 10 minutes a day writing a book and 10 minutes a day building a house that in a

174

couple of years, you would have saved a lot of money, you would speak a foreign language, would have written a book and built a house, all in under 40 minutes a day. I relate time management to the prospect sitting across from you during a sale. Every day you know you should do these things, but every day your mind tricks your body into "thinking about it," trying it out, into putting it off until the next day. That "other day" will never come. You will be an old person sitting around telling yourself, "I should have, I could have, if only..."

My mentor taught me one of the most valuable lessons I ever learned in this business. He said to me, "Have a five-year plan, have a one-year plan, have a monthly plan and have a daily plan." Looking back on it now, I did not always hit my daily plan. But I came pretty close. I did not always hit my monthly plan, but I came pretty close. I did not always hit my annual plan, but I would come pretty close. I think you know the answer to the five-year plan: If you can hit small goals, you can hit large goals. Take baby steps. No step is too small, and no goals or dreams are too big. If the dream has a plan and time is managed, anything can be accomplished. There are several books that have been written on time management. There are certainly several self-help books and movies as well. *Seven Habits of Highly Affective People* is one book that I recommend you should read.

There are two ways to work. You can work hard or you can work smart. I found the later to be much more lucrative.

My whole system is based on accountability to time management. The system can only work if you use it, and you can only use it if you manage your time correctly. Sit down with your manager or mentor and put together your goals. When you have done that, then work to devise a plan to achieve those goals. In the end, anything can be achieved.

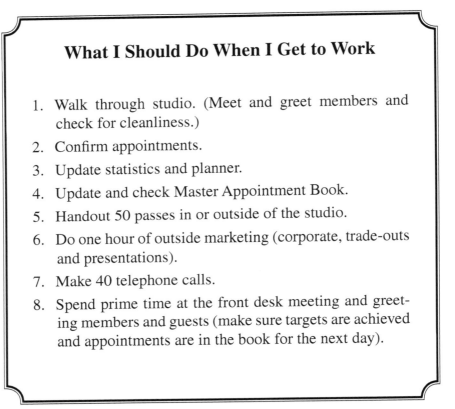

What I Should Do When I Get to Work

1. Walk through studio. (Meet and greet members and check for cleanliness.)

2. Confirm appointments.

3. Update statistics and planner.

4. Update and check Master Appointment Book.

5. Handout 50 passes in or outside of the studio.

6. Do one hour of outside marketing (corporate, trade-outs and presentations).

7. Make 40 telephone calls.

8. Spend prime time at the front desk meeting and greeting members and guests (make sure targets are achieved and appointments are in the book for the next day).

Chapter 36

HIRING AND TRAINING

I have been hiring and training salespeople for years, and in my experience, hiring the right yoga counselor is a consistence challenge in any business. I still have times when I hire a person that I think has no chance of being successful in sales. I still have times when I think the person is going to be the best employee I ever hired, and they turn out to be a poor yoga counselor and a poor employee. The reason this happens is that people behave different during an interview than they behave in real life. Just because someone gives a poor interview, does not make them a bad yoga counselor. Maybe it is that person's first interview, maybe the person is scared to death or maybe the person has not interviewed in years. It could also be that the person is nervous. Here is a list of questions you can ask that can help you improve your chances of hiring the right person.

Sample Interview Questions:

- Tell me a little bit about each one of your jobs in detail. What were your daily responsibilities? How long have you worked there and why did you leave?

- On a scale of 1 to 10, how important is making money? (If they do not care about making money, they will be tough to motivate.)

- What are your short-term goals? What are your long-term goals?

- Why do you see yourself as an advocate for yoga?
- At what level did you compete at organized or recreational sports?
- What would you do to get people to join our studios?
- How do you feel about rejection?
- When I call your ex-employers, what will they say were your strong points and/or your weak points?
- Have you ever been a member of a gym? If yes, tell me about your experience.
- How could you improve our yoga center? How could you improve our sales?
- What would you say if you try to sell me a membership and, after showing me all the prices, I say I will come back tomorrow or have to think about it?
- Have you ever sold anything before? On a scale of 1 to 10, how well did you do? And why did you leave?

I know there are a number of other great questions out there that can be used to ensure an effective interview. These are just a few that relate to our business, and you are welcome to use them. Remember, most of the time your first impression will be the right one. I have a good friend who works in human resources and, he hires people for a living. He tells me that his method is to hire everyone that he interviews and then eliminate the ones that do not perform. I do not know if I totally believe in this system, but I know that I definitely do not have a perfect way to tell you how to hire people. I can give you one word of advice, "Stay away from close friends and family members!" eventually you will, be put in a situation where you have to make a difficult decision about your friend or family member.

Remember, the more people you hire, train and mentor, the stronger the yoga counselor and manager you will become. You learn when you teach, and you will have a loyal student that will be there for you when you need them. You cannot move up in this business if you cannot replace yourself. You cannot manage more than one location without good managers working for you, and you cannot manage a studio without quality salespeople.

As buddy referrals work well with memberships, they also work well with the new hires.

Chapter 37

MAKING IT FUN

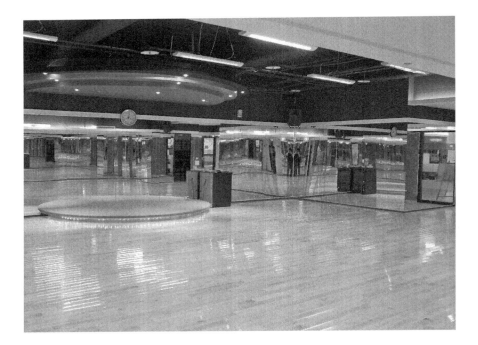

It is a yoga center, and it is supposed to be fun. Remember, although the yoga center business is still a business, you want to make sure that there is time to enjoy what we do. Many of the employees got into the business because of their love for yoga. So be sure that you include some crossover activities. You should have parties in your studio from time to time. You should have times during the day that you focus on having fun; for example, stop to play a game in the yoga room, have a contest or even some sort of yoga competition.

This may remind ex-athletes why they got into the yoga center business in the first place and this may help a new employee feel like a part of the team. Taking the staff out for a dinner or taking a trip to a local event can increase sales and moral. Every job has benefits and the business that we chose can be hard work and long hours but, if you put aside some time for your mental health your days as the complete yoga professional will be more productive and more enjoyable.

Chapter 38

MEMBER RETENTION

A lthough sometimes selling a membership seems like a war or you just played a mental game of chess, when the sale is closed and the membership is written up customer service and member retention are crucial. If your studios are like mine, your memberships are month to month, which means your member can cancel their monthly dues at any time. If you do not handle member retention correctly, you will watch your monthly dues base slide. Here are some easy steps to quality member retention.

Someone once told me the atmosphere at the front desk should be like Disneyland. Overly friendly!

Step 1

You must have a friendly front desk or service staff. Your customer service and front desk people have to be overly friendly. Do not hire anyone for these jobs who is not a happy, bubbly, outgoing person. They should be good on the telephones, courteous, wear huge smiles and make great eye contact. They should also say hello and goodbye to every member that enters the studio.

Step 2

You must have certified personal instructors that are available to offer free first workouts immediately following a member signing up. These individuals must look professional and call the new members to confirm the appointments. They must also be courteous to current members on the workout floor.

Step 3

The studio must be clean and spotless. The equipment must be maintained, and member complaints must be handled in a timely manner (lack of swift resolution of member complaints is the No. 1 reason for cancellations). Sometimes these members just want to vent, and when no one calls them back, they cancel.

Step 4

Call back all current members on a regular basis as a simple courtesy. Call all new members immediately after signing them up and welcome them to the studio.

These steps seem logical and are probably second nature to some of you already. You would be surprised to see how many studios do not follow these simple steps and pay for it in the end by having their members cancel or seeing their business drop.

Chapter 39

PRODUCTION MEETINGS

Production meetings are crucial to establishing accountability within the staff. Accountability is what drives production in a yoga center. With no accountability, nothing will get done. The production meetings should be short, ideally no more than 30 minutes. They should take place twice a day and should be positive and motivational. Goals should be set. Goals from the previous day should be checked. All guests and appointments should be tracked. Praises should be given, and the staff should be updated on promotions.

You have to "inspect what you expect." If you simply tell your salespeople to go handout passes, it will not get done. If you simply tell your salespeople to update their planners, it will not get done. If you simply tell your salespeople to update the master appointment book, it will not get done. The only way that it will get done is to say, "I want the master appointment book updated in the next 15 minutes, and I will be checking to see if it is done." Then after 15 minutes, follow through and check to see if it was updated. Create accountability. If you do not check, your staff will know that you do not follow through. They will, therefore, have no reason or motivation to update the master appointment book because they will know it will not be checked anyway, which equals no accountability.

The most productive operators in the business know how to handle all the issues in one meeting; this will free up the rest of the day for the important things like grossing.

In all the studios I operate, I set up a "war room." This room has two dry erase boards. One dry erase board is used to track the staffs' progress and create competition between them. The other board tracks the teams' progress. These two scoreboards will help your team understand the numbers and create healthy competition. I have put together a list called; "What a production meeting should look like." If you do this list daily, it will be almost impossible not to have a successful sales team.

What a Production Meeting should look like

- 11 am – All counselors and department heads should attend.
- All planners or appointment books should be checked and graded.
- All guest registers, TI's and the master appointment book should be checked from previous day. (Call back all missed guests.)
- All team members should have goals set for production and check goals from previous days' goals.
- Stats should be shared with everybody and a studio goal should be agreed upon and set.
- Role-play and training should be no more than 15 minutes.
- Motivate and update on promotions.

Good luck grossing!!!

Chapter 40

YOGA INSTRUCTORS

The yoga instructors in our studios today influence a larger group of members compared to any other employee in the yoga center. Don't you think it is time for the yoga centers to realize that 25 percent of all the people that come into our studios are there only to do yoga? They come in, they take a class and they leave. Think to yourself, how many of you are utilizing your yoga instructors for a source of revenue? Most yoga centers offer the classes free as part of the membership. I think in the yoga industry, this is the most underutilized department. Here are some ideas of how you can generate gross from your yoga instructors.

Please note that if you try to get older yoga instructors to do these things, it is going to be difficult. They are set in their ways, and they do not like change. Just like every other department in the studio, I recommend hiring and training your own instructors from scratch. That way they will know no other way than the way that you teach them (the right way, the productive way).

Step 1

Have your yoga instructors attend your production meetings. Update them on the specials and closeout sales. Then, in the beginning of each of their classes, they can make an announcement, talking about the discounts, savings the studio is offering and more. You may want to attend some of the classes yourself to make sure these important announcements are being made. This is a perfect time for a large group of people to hear wonderful things about your studio from somebody that they trust or admire.

Step 2

I like to have all of our yoga instructors wearing retail from our studio. This will help production in our clothing and retail department. You can even offer bonuses to yoga instructors that refer new memberships to your sales department.

Step 3

You can have your yoga instructors give a seminar in the beginning of class about weight loss. This can help you in sales of nutrition supplements or nutrition programs. And lastly, they can promote the benefits of supplementation. If you are a yoga counselor, you want to make sure that you are using your yoga instructors to increase your sales and have a continual source of upgrades, referrals, prepays, renewals and ancillary revenue. If you are the only yoga counselor in the studio using this most valuable resource, you are on the right track.

Chapter 41

THE BEST STUDIOS HAVE THE BEST TEAMS

I like to compare the yoga center business to sports teams. The reason why is that a lot of employees in yoga centers are athletes, and almost every person working in yoga has competitive attitudes because of their experience in athletics. Most sales force are driven by competition, the ability to hit certain goals, repetition and practice similar to playing a sport. As it is true in sports, I feel that the yoga center business is highly competitive. The teams with the best players, and the ability to work together, along with a skilled general manager will bring the most victories and most goals reached. I like to build my own teams from inexperienced salespeople, so they learn to work together. They have no bad habits, and they can learn at the same level. Sometimes when you hire experienced salespeople (go find hired guns) they don't meld with the rest of staff. They have different agendas, different techniques and can make new salespeople feel inferior. **"Remember, momentum is a large part of our business."** One staff member can ruin that momentum by causing controversy in the studio. Some salespeople thrive on the controversy. They intentionally cause problems, which causes the staff to get involved in solving the problem while they focus on their personal sale. This kind of cancer should be removed immediately. Sharks, controversial employees, non-team players and negative people will destroy any momentum that can be created by your team.

Together!!!

Everybody!!!

Achieves!!!

More!!!

"Inhale and God approaches you. Hold the inhalation,
and God remains with you. exhale, and you approach God.
Hold the exhalation, and surrender to God." - Krishnamacharya

Make sure praises are always given in public and reprimands are always given in private. Remember, it is a proven fact that your employees are happy at a company because of their ability to be recognized and feel good about their job. This is much more important than their financial rewards they receive. A good job at the end of the day can always take the place of a big raise.

Chapter 42

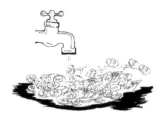

THE DUES BASE

Most salespeople do not fully understand what a "dues base" is or the beauty of what it does for your company. Some of the larger yoga center companies do not even explain to their managers what a dues base is or the amount of revenue that is brought in every month by the recurring monthly income known as the dues base. In short, the dues base is the monthly amount that is paid by the member to keep their membership active. It is collected in full from every member in the studio that did not pre-pay. Fifty members paying $25 a month means the studio's monthly dues base is $1,250 (50 members x $25). You should understand that for every member that prepaid, the company receives no residual income from that member. Yet the yoga center is still responsible for providing service.

For Example:

- If you sign up 30 members in 30 days, and they pay $1,000 for a three-year membership, you do that for one year, and at the end of that year, you will still need to sell 30 $1,000 memberships to hit a goal of $30,000.

- If you sell 30 one-year memberships that cost $25 a month, each month your dues base will increase $750 from those monthly payments alone. At the end of one year, if you were to sell 30 three-year memberships for $1,000, you will bring in $39,000 dollars. You have made more money for the studio selling memberships that are less expensive. The reason why is because you have $9,000 a month coming in from your monthly recurring dues. At this rate, in three years, you will be bringing in $27,000 a month without selling a membership.

This is the beauty of our business. For every dues membership we sell, we add to our monthly income. One of the problems in the yoga center industry today is that large yoga center company managers are unaware of what a dues base is. In a rush to get quick money, they take all of the monthly dues paying members and flip them into prepaid memberships, thinking that the immediate money will do them some good. You have to think about the future and keep the dues base active. For example, if a person is paying $39 a month and you tell them if they pre-pay for one year, you will give them one year for free. At that point, your studio will no longer receive that $39 monthly income, sacrificing it for a quick chunk of money. This practice is killing yoga centers, and it is killing any long- term yoga growth; therefore, it is killing yoga companies.

I know that large prepaid memberships are attractive. I know that collecting a large amount of money is a rush. I would recommend to any new yoga counselor or new manager that unless you are specifically told by your company or owner to sell prepaid memberships, that you focus your energy on selling at least 90 percent dues memberships. This will give your company the long-term stability to grow, to open new studios and to better the yoga industry as a whole.

The largest most successful companies in the world practice one common thing when it comes to billing. Monthly income is the key: gas companies, cable, telephone, electricity, insurance, banks and computers. The largest, most powerful companies in the world are built from their dues base.

Chapter 43

CLOSING SHEETS

A t the end of the night, most studios do a closing sheet. A closing sheet is the sheet used to update your stats for the next morning. The sheet may have a place for gross, EFT, closing percent and more. You can have your front desk person or closing person fill it out for you after the books have closed for that day. The closing sheet should be put in the manager's box so they do not have to try to find the information in the morning when it has already been sent to the corporate office. My general manager always wanted a copy of this sheet sent to his fax at the end of the night.

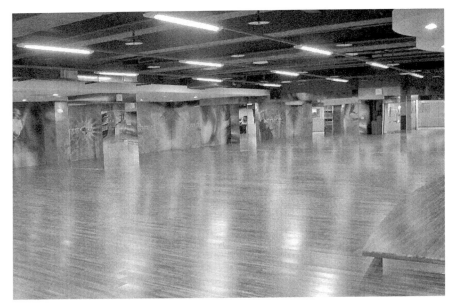

Selling Yoga

Closing Sheet

NMS (new membership sales) $_____

EFT (dues) $_____

RETAIL & DRINKS $_____

SUPPS $_____

OTHERS $_____

GUESTS $_____

DEALS $_____

TOTAL GROSS $_____

Please fax this sheet to the general manager at day's end.
(555-1212)

Chapter 44

ASKING QUESTIONS AND USING TIE DOWNS

I have found the art of yoga selling memberships is based mainly on asking questions to help our guests think for themselves and make their own decisions. You stimulate their thought process through a series of questions. It is important to let the guests answer the questions fully and completely before asking your next question. There is an old saying that goes, "telling is not selling." Wouldn't you agree? If you tell someone they need to lose weight or need to join the studio, they may believe you or they may doubt it. If you ask a person what brought them in today, and they say they need to lose weight, in that person's mind, it is true. The question, "What brought you in today?" stimulates the person to ask him or her, "Why *did* I come to the studio today?" After they answer your question, you may even want to follow up by asking, "Why do you want to lose weight?" They may answer, "My doctor told me I had to lose weight," or, "My clothes do not fit me anymore." At this point you may follow up that question by saying, "How does that make you feel?" These different questions will stimulate the guests to think on their own. It is important to let the guests make their own decisions based on their own thoughts. These thoughts can be stimulated through questions, not by statements and not by you telling them.

There is another practice that comes into play here. It is a little game that I invented and it has been instrumental in my success for training salespeople. The biggest mistake that new salespeople make comes in the form of answering all the guests' questions and using way too many statements. When they do this, the guests control the conversation and gains all of the information they need right then and there. They then tell the yoga counselor they need to think about it. Since there are no more questions to be asked, there is no more interest and there is no closing. The guests eventually leave without a membership in these situations. The game is called "the question game."

All of my new salespeople play this game for one hour a day during their first week of training. This game is instrumental in teaching the foundation and fundamentals of sales. A sale is a whole different way of talking and a whole different way of communicating. It is also totally unnatural. This game will help your new salespeople and yourself prepare for this difficult transition. The game is very simple, here is an example:

. Two salespeople sit face to face. The first yoga counselor asks a question. The other yoga counselor answers with a question, and so on and so forth. The key to the game is ignoring the question of the person sitting across from you and gaining control of the conversation by answering a question with another question. You may think this game sounds silly, but once you get good at it, you will understand the importance of "deaf earring."

"Deaf earring" means that many times your guests will ask questions, and they do not care about the response. This is simply a built-in defense mechanism used by your guests to stall and avoid commitment. If they really want to know the answer to the question, they will ask the question twice. You can even use words such as "by the way" to change the subject and regain the control of the conversation. Here is an example of the question game as an example. I will use 1. to signify person number one and 2. to person number two:

1. *"What time is the studio open?"* 2. *"What time will you be using the studio most?"*

1. *"How much is the membership?"* 2. *"Were you looking for yourself or someone else?"*

1. *"What kinds of yoga classes do you have?"* 2. *"What kinds of yoga classes are you interested in?"*

1. *"Do you have personal instructors?"* 2. *"Were you interested in a membership with one-on-one yoga or just a membership today?"*

As you can see, this game can come in handy. It will help you build the foundation and the fundamentals to increase sales and keep control of the conversation. The most important area that you will use this technique in is when you are filling out the membership agreement. This is the pivotal time when your guest is pulling out their credit card and trying to ask questions or stall. The right questions will keep you in control; they will isolate areas of interest and help you acknowledge facts. It is important to get minor agreement and arousal to increase emotional desire.

Another way we ask questions is to use something that we call a "tie down." A tie down is a question that usually ends with a guest giving a "yes" response. "Don't you agree?" "Sound fair?" "Don't you?" "Hasn't he?" "Wouldn't you?" "Won't you?" "Isn't it?" "Doesn't it?" You can even use tie downs at the beginning of a sentence to invoke a "yes" response. "Isn't the studio beautiful?" "Wouldn't you agree that we have everything you will need in order to accomplish your goals?" Remember to use tie downs sparingly because you will start to sound ridiculous if you use one at the end of every sentence.

Your first week as yoga counselor you should try a game I invented.
For one week answer every question asked with a question.
This will help you understand the fundamentals of sales!

Remember to use questions like who, what, when, were and why. It is important in sales to know how to answer questions by using your own questions in return. Tie downs will help you gain minor agreement from the guest. Asking the right questions will give you the information to customize a membership option to fit the most drastic needs of your guests.

Chapter 45

COMPENSATION PLANS

Finally, my paycheck! This area of the book can make a big difference in how much money you take home. It is important to understand exactly how you get paid. Most sales jobs pay a straight commission. You might be one of the lucky ones that have a base salary. I would like to take a moment to go over how you can maximize your commission.

- You must completely understand your compensation plan.

- You must ask as many questions as you can to clarify the "what if's."

- Sit down with the person that is signing the compensation plan and make notes (these will come in handy later).

- Remember that everything in this life is negotiable. (Do not think that just because it is in writing that it cannot be changed.)

- Make sure the plan includes job duties and responsibilities and also outlines holidays and working hours. (Since you work for a commission, you will be the first person asked to work over time.)

- You should understand how the rotation will work. How new leads will be allocated, and also the manner concerning "split" membership commissions will be implemented.

- The most important thing to understand is who your boss or people above you are.

- The last thing you want to know is what reasons would you be given a "no commission" on a membership (if there are a lot of reasons, go work somewhere else.)

Below, I have listed some of the vocabulary used in common compensation plans. This will outline some of the areas you will most likely be paid. Please be careful and ask some of the questions I have listed above. Remember, if you sign a long-term contract without first figuring out the details, you may be a very unhappy employee.

Base: The base salary is the money you receive for reporting to work and completing your daily responsibilities without making a sale.

Commission: The commission is a percentage of what you sell.

Draw: The draw is your company giving you a certain amount of money if you are unable to hit a certain number. For example, you have a $4,000 draw, and your sales commission only comes to $3,800, then the company will automatically give you the $4,000. Be careful. In some businesses, this money must be paid back from future checks.

Split: Is the percentage you receive when another yoga counselor sells your appointment.

No Commission: Some companies will pay no commission on a membership if the price is too low, incorrect or the membership agreement is not filled out properly.

Bonus: Bonus stands for a certain amount of money given if personal or studio objectives are met.

Residual Dues Base: Residual dues base is the amount of money coming in monthly from all the members you have signed up on monthly dues.

Percentage of Studio Gross: A percentage of all of the incoming money that the studio and the salespeople collect.

Percentage of New EFT: A percentage of all the new EFT collected by the studio or salespeople.

Goals: These are the goals set by your company for different areas of the studio.

Ancillary Revenue Commission: Ancillary revenue stands for vitamins, one-on-one yoga, nutrition, retail, tanning, massage and more.

401k or Medical and Dental programs: Benefits offered by the company to the employees

Family Memberships: Family memberships include the opportunity for employees to get discounts for their families or friends.

Profit Sharing *(make sure you are vested right away or don't get involved. You will be fired a week before you are vested)*: An opportunity for you to receive a portion of the company's profit, or an opportunity to be given a percentage of the company itself.

RTS: RTS stands for return to studio. It is for memberships that have not been filled out properly or need corrections or more signatures. (Make sure that you have a chance to fix any problems before being paid no commission.) Some companies will not give you this opportunity.

Chapter 46

PUT THE KIDS IN THE KID'S CLUB

I love kids, but if you don't learn how to make them work for you, the kids will work against you in the sales presentation. I am married and I have 3 children and I can certainly understand the priority that children have in a persons' life. I have been fortunate enough to set up my own business where I can spend two to three months a year vacationing and spending time with my family. To most parents, their kids are their Number one priority. If you can't learn to use the children to your advantage, they will hurt your odds of making a sale. If you come across a guest with children, you want to first focus on the children. Parents love to talk about their kids. Talk about the children and give the child a balloon. Get the child on your side. I always tell my new salespeople that they want to go into the child care and make the children feel comfortable. Stay in the child care with the parents, and outline the different services and options you have for the children. Whatever you do, don't just hand the child to the babysitter and walk away. If the kid starts crying, there is a good chance that you are going to miss the sale. I have even gone so far as to sell the entire membership inside the child care center. If a parent brings a child along on the tour, there is a good chance they will be bored and a parent will be distracted, therefore, not listening to the information they are receiving. Ultimately, they will use their child as an excuse that they are tired, bored or hungry, and they must leave.

Once the child is comfortable in the child care, (watching a movie and playing with other kids) then you can leave the child care area and sell your membership. Make sure that your presentation is brief. A young mother will not want to leave her child in the child care for very long. By the time you finish your tour, hopefully the child is well adapted and very happy in the child care center. If the child is not happy, then go ahead and sell the membership inside the child care center. If the child is happy, they will be your best ally. Nothing will help you to sell a membership more than a child who is having so much fun in your child care that they don't want to leave. I believe in increasing my sales percentages in all areas. Remember, it is a proven fact that women and families spend more money in a yoga center than any other demographic. The Ronald McDonald Play land has helped sell millions of hamburgers and the happy meal is the No. 1 selling fast food meal in America. McDonald's has used children to become one of the most successful chains of fast food restaurants using an average product. Use the children to your advantage, and you will increase your percentages and help mothers and families create a healthful lifestyle.

Chapter 47

BUDDY REFERRALS

If you listen to any old-time yoga salesmen, they will tell you that the lifeblood of the yoga industry is buddy referrals (BRs). In some ways, I still believe this to be true. Of the numerous studios that I have been blessed to work in we sold more memberships from buddy referrals than from any other lead source. I have attached the BR cards we presently use; feel free to use it, or change it to fit your personal needs. The card has several key areas.

- You explain to a member that it is a VIP pass only given to new members.

- There must be a deadline date, two to three days, where their buddy must pick up the pass.

- There should be an area for only a few names and telephone numbers (more than two or three spaces make the pass seem invaluable).

- The pass should be anywhere from one week to one month in length.

- The member must understand the value of the VIP pass.

- You should explain to the member that this pass also allows their buddies to receive the same membership price as them for 30 days from the time you enroll.

- My studio offers a promotion that if you bring five new members to the studio to join within 30 days, they will receive one year for free. (Must be the same price or higher).

If the new member gives you the name and the number of a friend, you should call them immediately and let them know that you have a two-week free membership waiting for them and that they have only 48 hours to validate their passes.

VIP Guest Membership

As a valued new member, you can place family members, friends, acquaintances and business associates on your VIP guest list so they can receive a free two-week VIP trial membership. In order to qualify, they must be listed on your VIP guest list. There is absolutely no obligation for anyone that you refer. We will simply present the two-week membership as a gift from you. All two-week memberships must be activated within 48 hours from the date of enrollment.

For example:

Your Personal Information (please print)

Name _____ Date _____ / _____ / _____

Home Phone _____ Cell Phone _____

Work Phone _____

Employer _____

Does your company provide any employee yoga incentives?

_____ Yes _____ No

Name	Home Phone	Business Phone
1. _____	_____	_____
2. _____	_____	_____
3. _____	_____	_____

Who can I make a V.I.P. Guest

Friends, relatives, acquaintances, business associates or any-one you think would enjoy receiving a gift of a two-week free VIP membership. When you think about it, just about anyone can benefit from staying fit. Do not wait and risk having one of your guests pay a guest fee when you can give them a free VIP membership. Any member who refers five memberships of equal price or more within 30 days of enrollment will receive one year free.

Chapter 48

INCREASE YOUR SALES KNOWLEDGE

As the complete professional, you must continue to grow. You must improve your knowledge, your sales skills and your training information. Our business is a rapidly changing one. If you do not continue to grow, you will be left in the dust. The young people just starting in our business are at the top of their game. They are top athletes trained by the latest technology, and they know there is money to be made in our industry. They are hungry. There is a poster above my desk and it says,

"Every morning on the planes of Africa, the lion awakes, and knows it must outrun the slowest gazelle or it will starve to death. Every morning on the same plane, the gazelle awakes and knows it must outrun the fastest lion, or it will be killed." It does not matter if you are the lion or the gazelle. When you wake up in the morning, you'd better be running."

We work in the one of the fastest growing industries in the world. Computerization has changed the amount of energy that we expel at work. By the year 2010, 25 percent of all Americans will be working from their homes. You literally will not even have to get up and walk in order to accomplish your job. The obesity rate is reaching staggering numbers. The amount of information about yoga changes every day. Doctors are getting smarter. Nutritionists are getter better. Supplementation has improved. Lets face it yoga centers have come a long way from the old strap machine that jiggles your fat away (by the way, there was still one of those in the first gym that I worked).

Selling Yoga

"Anyone who practices can obtain success in yoga but not one who is lazy constant practices is the secret of success."
- Hatha Yoga Pradipika

My mentor once told me that there are two kinds of people in this business. There is the rock, and there is the sponge. The rock can sit in the water forever, and the water cannot penetrate it. The rock remains dry inside. Then there is the sponge. The sponge, when put in the water absorbs, it grows in size and weight. We can use this analogy to describe the two types of professionals in our business. The information is the water. For the rock, the information will never penetrate: They already know everything. They do not have the humility to accept change. Then there is the sponge. The person who is the sponge is able to absorb new information. The professional grows in size and skill and willingness to try new things with the humility to accept new information. I recommend attending as many seminars as you possibly can. I also recommend reading the latest information about our trade. Take this information, test it, try it and improve it.

Chapter 49

DRILLING

Practice makes perfect. Drilling is an essential part of the human behavioral learning process. Repetition is the key to perfection. Doing things over and over is the key to perfection. Each time it is done, we improve just a little bit more. Until we can do it without even thinking, this is the place that we long to be. The unconscious competence: You don't have to think about riding a bike, and you don't have to think about catching a ball. You don't have to think about walking. But all of these things at one point in our life were difficult. It took a lot of effort and practice to perfect these simple things.

Selling is no more difficult than riding a bike. The sales trade may be difficult to a beginner, but in some ways it can be as easy as riding a bike. Most people at the age of five learn to ride a bike. They don't learn to sell. A professional football player practices throwing a football every day of his life and still continues to practice every day once he gets in the pros. All professional's drill: boxers, basketball players, racecar drivers, doctors and lawyers. Practice, practice, practice, drill, drill, drill.

Mirroring and Matching Drill

This drill requires two counselors sitting face to face mirroring and matching every movement. You want to focus on the energy, the breathing, everything involved in mimicking the person to a "T."

The Question Game

The question game is a simple but effective way to master the art of selling. This technique has been instrumental in my ability to train top-notch yoga sales professionals. Answering a question with a question and staying calm under fire is at the heart of what selling is all about. It took me a long time to develop a drill that could teach the fundamentals that were the real difference between a new sales person and a seasoned one. One day it dawned on me that the difference between a new sales person and a seasoned was as simple as the experienced professional knowing how to ask questions instead of answering them. This is the little or **big** difference in communication styles! This drill helped put the salesperson in control of the conversation thus enabling them to control the thoughts of the guest through a series of questions. When each of the questions is asked the guest needs time to think of the answer and the sales process begins. This drill is my invention and I have never seen it used in any other publication. To perform the drill, sit across from another yoga counselor and ask them a question. The other counselor (in a role playing manner), will then answer with a question, to which you will reply with another question and so forth.

Example:

Yoga Counselor 1: How much does it cost for a one on one yoga training package?

Yoga Counselor 2: Were you looking for a training package for yourself, a family or a couple?

Yoga Counselor1: Do you have any Pilates classes?

Yoga Counselor 2: What kind of Pilates classes are you interested in?

Yoga Counselor 1: Do you have a sauna?

Yoga Counselor 2: Were you interested in a yoga membership with use of the sauna or just a membership today?

Yoga Counselor 1: What time is the studio the busiest?

Yoga Counselor 2: What time will you be using the studio most?

Repetition is the mother of learning and the father of action, which makes it the architect of accomplishment

The Tough Customer Drill

This is a great drill for new yoga counselors. You have to learn to be direct and to come back at your guest with the same energy they are giving you. This is not the time to back down. Your guest is trying to take control. This is their technique. This is the time for you to take control by matching the abrasiveness brought on by your rude guest.

Closing Drill

In a role-playing situation, try to overcome objections given by your manager or another yoga counselor. Ask your partner, "If I can get you a great deal on a membership, would you want to get started today?" Have your partner respond by saying, "Not today, maybe, I want to try it first, I would consider it and no." Drill on overcoming these objections. You may try "if it was $20 a year, you wouldn't join the studio today?" Also drill on "out of the different membership options, which one are you leaning towards?" Your partner would respond with the eight common objections. "I want to think about it!" "I need to speak to my spouse." "It is too much money." Use the steps outlined in overcoming objections. Practice overcoming five objections, and make sure your partner is being realistic: not too hard, and not too easy.

Tough Telephone Inquiry (TI) drill

Role-play on a difficult TI caller. Practice using the telephone inquiry script. Perfect the art of leaving no space between your questions and the callers' answers. Learn to control conversations. Practice using the script verbatim. Your partner should consistently try to ask price. Remain calm and answer questions with questions. For example, say, "How much is a membership?" "How did you hear about the studio?" "How much is a membership?" "Are you looking for yourself or you and someone else?" "Can't you just give me the price?" "I would love to answer all of your questions, but I just need a little information, what are your main yoga goals?"

Filling out the Membership Agreement Drill

This is probably the most important drill, and this is probably the area where most new sales counselors lose their guests or miss their sales. Practice stalling tactics. Practice grabbing the membership agreement. Practice answering questions with questions. Practice tapping your finger at the signature spot. Bring up objections over EFT. Bring up objections about payment method or type. Bring up objections about coming back to pay later. If you can perfect through practice, the ability to control your guest during this most important time in the sales process, you will find this will highly increase your closing percentages.

One-on-one Yoga Presentation

Practice your P.T. presentation learn it word for word. Drill on your guest asking difficult detailed questions on yoga. Your presentation should sound smooth and unrehearsed. You should practice being an empathetic listener and your presentation should build value in the program.

Seven Most Common Objections Drill

Outline the seven most common objections. Try to overcome them as fast as possible. This drill is designed to get the right answer quickly and smoothly.

Chapter 50

CORPORATE MEMBERSHIPS

Selling a corporate membership can be a great way to generate new members and increase your personal paycheck. This avenue can be a reliable source of gross. Your company can benefit tremendously from memberships created from companies that are looking for healthful benefits for their employees. The key to a successful corporate relationship will start with a well thought out plan and knowledge of what will work and what will not work. As long as I have been in the yoga center business, I have seen thousands of new yoga counselors that had some idea of producing 500 memberships that would be the direct result of a corporate account. Trust me. I don't waste time on things that are not proven, although I do like to try new things. But to be honest, most of what I see are new yoga counselors trying things that have been proven to be ineffective. Remember that selling a corporate membership will be different than the emotional sale made at the table in your office.

Six Important Steps to Remember When Selling a Corporate Membership

1. You must be a professional. The old sweat pants may not work in the corporate office at IBM.

2. Understand that large companies allocate funds for their employees and that money must be spent. The relationship or personal benefit to the contact person may be the thing that closes the deal.

3. Most corporate deals take time. The relationship between the company and your yoga centers must be a symbiotic one. Take a long-term approach to offering all yoga needs to the company. You must be available to offer your services. This may include health fairs, board meetings, progress reports, demonstrations and information on corporate savings through health.

4. Companies have agendas. Most decisions are made by a group. The more information you can provide indicating the corporation will save money and add production, the better your chances of a large paycheck.

5. Keep any studies on companies that have been successful in improving their production through promoting yoga or have lowered sick days through wellness.

6. Be careful to make sure that you make appointments for all employees so they are given proper service at the studio. You don't want the decision maker to come in on your day off and get pounded by the shark in your studio.

Common Concerns of the Corporate Account

- What if my employees don't use the studio?
- How will the benefits outweigh the cost?
- Why your company?
- Can your company show our company the benefits or end results?
- Can you offer something that doesn't cost us?
- Can you offer something that doesn't cost us if the employee's don't use the studio or get results?

The Options

1. The company offers to pay the enrollment fee. Each of the employees can then handle the monthly dues. This gives the employee the option to enroll with a discount.

2. The company pay's for one-year membership at a discount; an example is 10 employees for $399; 20 employees for $349; 40 employees for $299; or 60 or more employees $229.

3. The company buys bulk passes, one-day workouts. Every time an employee uses the facility they simply present the pass. (These work well for the employer that has a concern that their staff may not use the studio.) Bulk passes also work great for employee incentives. (100 at $8 per pass; 200 at $7 per pass; 300 at $6 per pass; 1000 at $4 per pass 2,000 or more at $3 per pass)

4. You may try a sign-in list where the company pays a set amount per sign in, at the end of each month.

5. The most popular way of offering a discount to a company would be to us the old corporate flyer. This approach would in no way obligate the company. Simply put the flyer up by the company time clock or in the lunch room, and their employees can enroll at the studio at a discounted rate. (Be sure as with everything to add urgency, with an enrollment period or an expiration date.)

Employees of Home Depot Corporate Discount
Huge Savings off the Regular Rate

Enrollment	~~399~~	0
Processing		49
Monthly Investment		25

Ask for Mary   Tel:555-1212

Hurry ! Expires 1/1/08

Must show corporate ID at time of enrollment, must be valid age. Some restrictions apply, family members can add on at the point of sale for an additional 19 dollars per month

---

Chapter 51

THE SALES PROFESSIONAL CODE

As the complete sales professional it is important to grade your-self in an honest manner. Self-reflection is a way of making sure that the product that you are selling remains the primary focus. As you grow and fully understand the sales process you will begin to internalize and understand that in most cases the product that you are selling is **YOU**. Once you understand this rule, you will begin to develop a system of improving the product. Below I have outlined a detailed code of daily affirmation. That will aid in your healthy relationship between your trade and your life.

1. I am human and I am a slave to my daily routine.

   My daily routine attacks my free will, due to years of accu-mulative habits and the past deeds of my life. I have already marked a path which threatens to imprison my future. My ac-tions are ruled by my appetite, passion, prejudice, greed, love, fear, environment, and habit. And the worst of these tyrants is habits. I will form good habits and become their slave.

2. I will greet this day with love in my heart.

   My reasoning they may counter; my speech they my distrust; my apparel they may disapprove; my face they may reject; and even my bargains may cause them suspicion; yet my love will melt all hearts liken to the sun whose rays soften the coldest clay.

3. I will persist till I succeed.

    I am a lion and I refuse to talk, to walk, to sleep with the sheep. I will hear not those who are weak and complain, for their disease is contagious. Let them join the sheep. The slaughter house of failure is not my destiny. The prizes of life are at the end of each journey, not near the beginning.

4. I am nature's greatest miracle.

    I am rare, and there is value in all rarity; therefore, I am valuable. I am the end of product of thousands of years of evolution; therefore, I am better equipped in both mind and body than all the emperors and wise men that preceded me.

5. I will live this day as if it is my last.

    I will waste not a moment moaning yesterday's misfortune, yesterday's defeat, yesterday's heartache, for why should I throw away good after that. This is my day to excel.

6. Today I will be the master of my emotions.

    I will learn this secret of the ages: Weak is he who permits his thoughts to control his actions; strong is he who forces his actions to control his thoughts. Each day, when I awaken, I will follow this plan of battle before I am captured by the forces of sadness, self-pity and failure.

7. I will laugh at the world.

    I will laugh at my failures and they will vanish in clouds of new dreams; I will laugh at my success and they will shrink to their true value. I will laugh at evil and it will die untested;

I will laugh at goodness and it will thrive and abound. Each day will be triumphant only when my smiles bring the forth smiles.

8. Today I will multiply my value a hundredfold.

    I will set goals for the day, the week, the month, the year, and my life. Just as the rain must fall before the wheat will crack its shell and sprout, so must I have objectives before my life will crystallize. In setting my goals I will consider my best performance of the past and multiply it a hundredfold.

9. I will act now.

    My dreams are not worthy. My plans are nothing and my goals are impossible. All are of no value unless they are followed by action. Action is the good and the drink which will nourish my success. I must always act without hesitation and the flutters in my heart will vanish.

10. I shall have faith in my higher power.

    Never will I seek delivery of gold, love, good health, pretty victories, fame, success, or happiness. Only for guidance will I pray, that I may be shown the way to acquire these things, and my prayers will always be answered. The guidance I seek may come, or the guidance I seek my not come, but are not both of these an answer? I will pray for guidance.

OG MANDINO

Chapter 52

TO SELL OR NOT TO SELL

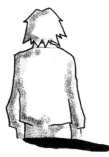

To sell or not to sell, that is the question. Recently, we have been hearing the faint whispers of a growing number of business professionals blaming the sales process as the smoking gun for all of the shortcomings in our industry. This negative force has been deemed the reason for some kind of slow growth. When putting some deep thought into this important issue we must look at our industry and we must look into the future as well as into the past. The first question I ask is "**what** slow growth?" The Yoga business next to the size of the McDonalds coke may be the fastest growing thing on the planet. Due to the present down turn in the economy most companies within our core markets failed to survive. While all the other businesses are thinking of ways to improve and enhance the sales process we are thinking of abandoning it.

The shortcomings that we have are a staple in any growing business. Ours comes not from the selling process but more from the lack of getting all of our ships to sail in the same direction. Not in the selling process but in the professional level, or lack thereof, which our industry requires for training and keeping a mature staff. Selling is a tool and nothing more "should the chef stop creating his mastery's in the kitchen because he is burned by the flame or blame the knife for a nick on the finger?"

Selling is a tool and when used properly it may be referred to as the greatest profession ever created by man! However, it is a very powerful and complicated tool, when used properly it can be extremely effective and when used carelessly it can be dangerous. Studied in depth it is as powerful and infinite as the human mind and yet it is also as basic in human nature as children's first questions. I agree our process must evolve and it will, but it must do so without abandoning the knowledge gained by our predecessors.

We must understand that we are dealing with people as our product. We sell dreams and results and sometimes failure, thus we must endeavor to understand that each and every guest is different. We must also accept that the incredible growth of our industry could be called the most explosive business invention of the century.

To those who say this industry and its systems are not extra ordinary and that growth means the abandonment of competition, victory and selling dreams, I say never.

OTHER BOOKS
BY RON THATCHER
www.amazon.com

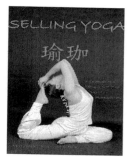

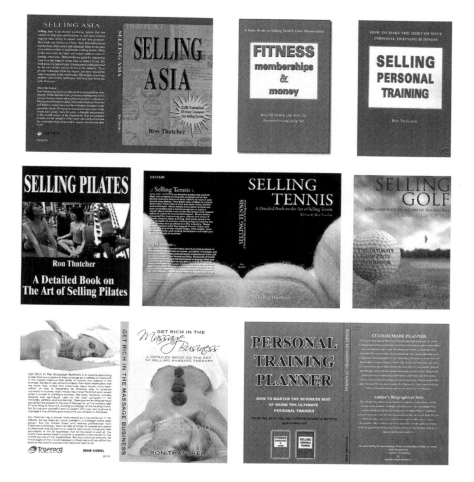

FAST & EASY

www.fitnessjobpost.com

NO LOG-IN REQUIRED

www.fitnessjobpost.com

FREE 2 MONTH TRAIL FOR EMPLOYERS

www.fitnessjobpost.com

POST JOBS

SEARCH RESUMES

JOB SEEKERS-FREE

POST RESUMES

JOB ALERTS

www.fitnessjobpost.com

FAST EASY NO HASSLE #775-671-0521

Made in the USA
Lexington, KY
28 February 2010